ESSENTIAL NURSING CARE

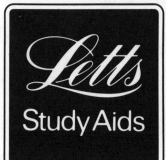

Letts Study Aids

Janet Clark BEd Hon, SRN, RCNT, DN (London), RNT
Senior Tutor, Avon School of Nursing, Bristol Royal Infirmary

Christine Sage MSc, SRN, SCM, MTD, RNT, TCert Ed
Senior Lecturer in Nursing Studies,
Polytechnic of the South Bank

Moira Attree MSc, BNurs, SRN, NDN, HV, RNT
Former Nurse Tutor, Manchester Royal Infirmary

D0185666

Charles Letts & Co Ltd
London, Edinburgh & New York

First published 1985
by Charles Letts & Co Ltd
Diary House, Borough Road, London SE1 1DW

Reprinted 1986

Revised 1988

Illustrations: Tek-Art and Kate Charlesworth

© J. E. Clark, C. A. Sage, M. J. Attree 1985, 1988
© Illustrations: Charles Letts & Co Ltd 1985, 1988

British library Cataloguing in Publication Data

Clark, Janet
    Revise essential nursing care ——
    Rev. ed —— (Letts study aids).
    I. Nursing
    I. Title   II. Sage, Christine   III. Attree, Moira
    610. 73   RT41

ISBN 0 85097 683 9

'Letts' is a registered trademark of
Charles Letts & Co Ltd

Printed and bound in Great Britain by
Charles Letts (Scotland) Ltd

Preface

This revision book for nurses is intended to provide a reasoned foundation for essential care using a problem solving approach, during the first year to eighteen months of training.

Assessment of patient problems is the foundation for care planning. Skills of observation, deduction and analysis are required to interpret findings and to plan and evaluate care. Each unit has been based upon a concept of normal activity of daily living or a fundamental physiological process, e.g. maintaining blood pressure. Care plans illustrate an 'anonymous' patient's care for a related medical condition which produces the 'problem'. The nurse must construct his/her own care plan, using the suggested plan as a guide only. Theory related to more than one unit will be required for patients with multiple problems.

Reading is suggested at the end of each chapter. Articles from journals are recommended which illustrate patients' problems. This book should be used in conjunction with the additional reading, and application can then be made to the patient in the ward or the community. Understanding why certain care is effective will improve reasoned decision making, improve practice and promote patient safety. Multiple choice questions to review each unit and two practice tests are set at the end of the book.

The authors are all widely experienced in the practice and teaching of nursing.

Acknowledgements

We would like to thank Charles Letts for providing the opportunity to write this book, and especially to thank editors Pat Rowlinson and Ruth Holmes for all their help and encouragement. Thanks also to Anne Davison who designed the book and Tek-Art and Kate Charlesworth for the illustrations. Typing of the manuscript was undertaken by the authors and Christine and Marjorie to whom we are grateful. Last but not least a thank you to husband John and friends for their untiring support.

Janet Clark
Christine Sage

January 1985

Contents

Section I

Introduction

Since 1948 the health of this country has been taken care of by the now massive machinery of the National Health Service. Many would argue that the word 'sickness' should be used rather than 'health'. This is because the service that is provided is geared towards making sick people well rather than towards the prevention of sickness. Thus the money is spent on modern technology, for example, rather than providing a full annual health check for everyone which can serve not only to detect early signs of disease but also to teach people how to live healthy lives.

This large and complex organization is run by teams of managers at varying levels often represented in the shape of a triangle with nurses like yourselves at the base of this triangle next to the patients whom the whole seeks to serve. Those at the bedside often doubt the caring of the managers as they are left to cope with the shortages and difficulties particularly in times of economic recession. Sometimes the nurse feels frustrated because she cannot give the level of care that she would like because of the pressure of work. Sometimes frustration is increased because of the feeling of being unable to influence the system.

However, it is the most junior nurses who are closest to the patients and to whom the patient most frequently turns for help, comfort and to answer their questions. It is still the student nurse rather than the trained nurse who carries out most of the basic nursing care and therefore the standard of nursing care is often set by the students. This book aims to help you set not only safe but caring standards. The UKCC have set a Code of Professional Conduct in which they set out the standards that they expect all trained nurses to maintain; failure to do so could lead to disciplinary action. (See Appendix, page 147). As a revision book it does not have all the answers but it does contain most of the relevant underlying principles which you can apply to specific situations. This book then is seen to complement the rich resources you will find in your own training school. Do make use of your personal tutor who will be pleased to discuss issues and help you with your studies.

From 1986–88 onwards Registered General Nurse students will be assessed on the competencies (b) to (h) given by the United Kingdom Central Council training rule 18 (see below)

Courses leading to a qualification the successful completion of which shall enable an application to be made for admission to Part 1 of the register shall provide opportunities to enable the student to accept responsibility for her personal professional development and to acquire the competencies required to:

(a) advise on the promotion of health and the prevention of illness;

(b) recognize situations that may be detrimental to the health and well-being of the individual;

(c) carry out those activities involved when conducting the comprehensive assessment of a person's nursing requirements;

(d) recognize the significance of the observations made and use these to develop an initial nursing assessment;

(e) devise a plan of nursing care based on the assessment with the co-operation of the patient, to the extent that this is possible, taking into account the medical prescription;

(f) implement the planned programme of nursing care and where appropriate teach and co-ordinate other members of the caring team who may be responsible for implementing specific aspects of the nursing care;

(g) review the effectiveness of the nursing care provided, and where appropriate, initiate any action that may be required;

(h) work in a team with other nurses, and with medical and para-medical staff and social workers;

(i) undertake the management of the care of a group of patients over a period of time and organize the appropriate support services;

related to the care of the particular type of patient with whom she is likely to come in contact when registered in that Part of the register for which the student intends to qualify.

This book aims to help the student develop these competencies and so successfully complete her training.

There are some concepts that are explicit or implicit in much of the text. Rather than repeating ourselves we have decided to deal with them here in the Introduction.

'Reassure the patient'

This is a cliché frequently used by nurses when describing the care they would give a patient exhibiting signs of anxiety, but how are you to accomplish this? As soon as a person becomes aware of a difficulty, for example difficulty in breathing, they also become aware of a feeling of rising panic. They may be well aware that to give in to the panic will make the situation worse. Have you ever tried to control rising panic? If the situation is short-lived you may succeed; but if not, few people can remain in control without someone to help. Often the very presence of another person may be sufficient, particularly if that person seems quietly in control of the situation. If your immediate 'first aid' steps work, this will increase the patient's confidence in you. Be sure to listen to the patient, not only to his or her words, but to the very powerful non-verbal communications. The patient's fear and agitation will be increased if he or she feels that you are not listening and understanding.

For many people information regarding what is going on now, and what will happen next, goes a long way towards reducing stress (Hayward, 1975; Boore, 1978).

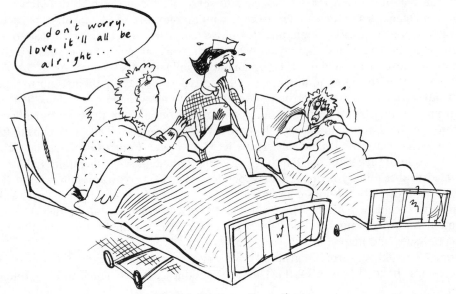

Fig. I.1 Reassure the patient

Teaching patients

Part of our role as nurses is to teach patients. This teaching may be of a general nature as in the principle of living a healthy life, or more specific as in teaching a patient a specific skill, e.g. giving their own injections or re-education in the performing of any one of the activities of daily living. The following general points on the learning process may help you in your teaching activities.

1 *Prepare the patient*:
   Ensure that they are not over-tired.
   Ensure that they have no immediate needs (thirsty – hungry – need to eliminate).
   Ensure that they are comfortable.

2 *Arouse interest*:
   Show how the activity will aid their recovery.
   Prepare appropriate 'visual aids'.
   Perhaps involve a patient who has already learnt the skill.

3 *Material must be meaningful*:
   Appropriate use of language.
   Be sure to explain specialist terms.

4 *Material must have*:
   A pattern.
   A logical sequence.

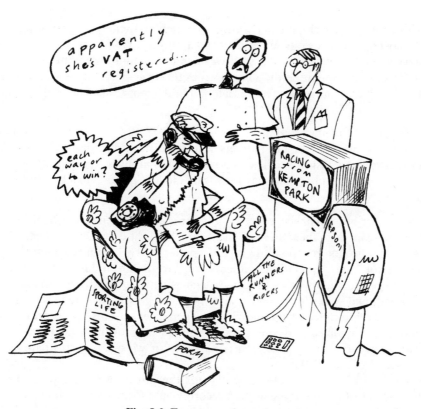

Fig. I.2 Encourage the patient

5 *Pace yourself*:
   Too fast – results in despair.
   Too slow – results in frustration.

6 *Repeat the exercise*:
   As often as necessary.
      BUT
   Beware not to over-tire the patient.
   Learning may take a very long time but remember that practice makes perfect.

7 *Give plenty of 'rewards'*:
   Encourage the patient.
   Praise each small step of advance.

Be sure to set realistic goals. This requires a careful analysis of the subject or skill you wish to teach. When we master a skill it becomes a habit and we are rarely conscious of the steps we have taken to accomplish the task. Take, for example, tying shoe laces, or giving an injection, or even driving a car; until we acquire the skill it all seems so complex. How can I look in the mirror, steer and change gear at the same time?

The teaching of the simplest task can take patients a very long time, particularly if there is neuro-muscular involvement. Patients have to re-learn how to control the affected muscles before they can begin to perform the task; this in itself is tiring. We therefore need to be very patient and understanding. Frustation and anger may be exhibited by patients. This may be the time to stop the lesson temporarily, encourage an entirely different pursuit, or a rest as appropriate, before returning to the learning activity a little later.

Communication

This is a two-way process and consists of:

1 Listening
2 'Speaking'

Speaking is in quotation marks because we can speak using words – verbal communication – or using our bodies – non-verbal communication. When assessing patients, questioning may form a major part of the interview process. Worksheets to develop the skills of questioning are to be found in the Appendix, page 149. Body language is very powerful and most people will respond to the non-verbal cues when there is dissonance between verbal and non-verbal messages. When we approach patients are we approaching them as equals or as superiors? I suspect that most of us convey our superiority and authority. Why? Because often patients are in bed and we stand by the bed to speak. If we wish to communicate with them as equals we should sit to ensure that we are at the same level as they are. This will also encourage eye-to-eye contact. However, a nurse can feel threatened in this position as her vulnerability can be revealed. Menzies (1970) states that:

'Nurses are in constant contact with people who are physically ill . . . the recovery of the patients is not certain. . . . Nursing patients who have incurable diseases is one of the nurse's most distressing tasks. . . . The work situation arouses very strong and mixed feelings in the nurse: pity, compassion, and love, guilt, anxiety, hatred, and resentment. . . .'

Menzies then describes what she calls socially structured defence mechanisms which are employed to help cope with these stresses. An example of these would be the mechanism that ensures the nurses do not get too close to their patients. This would include having several patients to care for, and changing the patients you care for from day to day. These defence mechanisms are reinforced by other processes such as depersonalization both of patients (the paraplegic in bed) and staff (the second-year nurse); categorization (medical/surgical patient) and denial of the significance of the individual. These mechanisms act to prevent any nurse from becoming too involved with one patient; they also unfortunately militate against real communication, and real communication is necessary if we are to aid a patient's recovery (Hayward, 1975; Boore, 1978).

Communication in writing is also essential for the nurse. All nursing records are legal documents. In cases of litigation the written record would form an important part of the legal proceedings. Failure to record nursing care could lead to disciplinary action (See UKCC Code of Professional Conduct–Appendix, page 147). Examples of suggested care plans are therefore included to help you develop competence.

This book, then, is about essential nursing care. It attempts to keep the patient central, recognizing individual differences and therefore individual needs. At the same time it recognizes that nurses are inclined to talk in clichés. The authors have, therefore, not only made every effort not to fall into this trap, but to give examples of what such clichés mean in practice. The book is aimed primarily at junior nurses. It sets out to equip them with the essential information that is required to ensure safe practice. It does not, however, pretend to be a complete nursing text. It is a very practical book and its main aim is to help build up a nurse's confidence in her daily interactions with her patients.

Most of the units are based around the type of problem with which a patient may present, for example, a problem with mobility, or with breathing. Some of the units do not quite fit into this model but were included because the authors felt, from their experience with students/pupils, that they were areas that many found difficult to handle–for example, care of the dying.

The Appendix includes useful data that are not normally available within one volume but to which students may need to refer. The comprehensive sets of questions should help the student or pupil to learn the material, making her a better practitioner and a successful examination candidate.

References
Boore, J. R. P. *Prescription for Recovery* (Churchill Livingstone, 1978)
Hayward, J. *Information and Prescription Against Pain* (RCN, 1975)
Menzies, I.E.P., *The functioning of social systems as a defence against anxiety* (The Tavistock Institute of Human Relations, 1970).

Section II Core units 1–11

1 The promotion of health

1.1 Promotion of health

The promotion of health is accepted as a fundamental role of all nurses. As we saw on page 1 the UKCC training rule 18(a) states that general nurses shall be competent to:

'advise on the promotion of health . . .'

The International Council of Nurses places the promotion of health as the first of their four-fold responsibilities of a nurse.

1.2 Definitions of health

Before we can discuss how we are to promote health we need to decide what we mean by health. To a certain extent the concept of health is specific to the individual. Each individual has his own view which will affect his perception of himself, his relationship to others and his environment, and his goals and values in life. Thus a person with a physical handicap may consider himself healthy as long as the handicap does not cause generalized problems. Despite the difficulties in defining what we mean by health, a working definition is useful, if somewhat inadequate. According to the World Health Organization (WHO) health is:

'A state of complete physical, mental, and social well-being, not merely the absence of disease or infirmity.' (WHO, 1947)

The same body went a step further at their 30th Assembly in 1977 by declaring:

'The attainment by all citizens of the world by the year 2000, of a level of health that will permit them to lead a socially and economically productive life.' (WHO, 1977)

1.3 Promoting independence and the feeling of well-being

One method of analysing the interaction that occurs between people is to use transactional analysis. In itself it does not give us a complete picture, but it may help us to understand a little of what may happen between us and our colleagues and patients. Such an understanding may help us to promote independence and the feeling of well-being. One of the earliest exponents of this method of analysis was Eric Berne. Each human being has, according to Berne (1961), three aspects to his personality which influence his everyday action. These three aspects are called three ego states (an ego state is defined as a consistent pattern of thinking, feeling or behaving). Berne refers to these three states as the parent, adult and child (see Fig. 1.1). We all have these three aspects to our personality. Sometimes one is uppermost, sometimes the other. A well-balanced adult will spend most of the time in the adult state. However, when we are sick we are all inclined to regress to the child state. We want to be looked after and have decisions taken for us, that is as long as the decisions made for us prove to be the right ones.

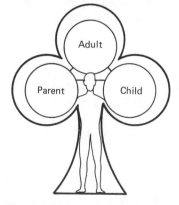

Fig. 1.1 Transactional analysis

For fundamentals of transactional analysis see Villière (1981). Figs. 1.2 and 1.3 show how transactional analysis illustrates the effectiveness of communication.

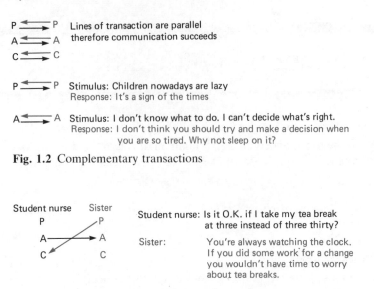

Fig. 1.2 Complementary transactions

Lines of transaction are crossed, therefore communication breaks down.

Fig. 1.3 A crossed transaction or 'game'

Crossed transactions can result in the patient, medical staff and nurses being caught up into what Berne (1964) refers to as a game. Games provide benefits to all players in that they protect the integrity of the position without the threat of uncovering the position. However, every game is basically dishonest and the outcome has a dramatic quality. Games, according to Villière (1981), promote lower achievements, poor morale, hurt feelings, distrust and poor communications. Thus if medical staff and nurses are prepared to play this game then they must be prepared to accept the anger that will be hurled at them if things go wrong.

Virginia Henderson (1965) said that nursing was:

'. . . primarily helping people, sick or well, in the performance of those activities contributing to health, or its recovery (or to a peaceful death) that they would perform unaided if they had the necessary strength, will or knowledge . . . to help people gain independence as rapidly as possible.'

Thus Henderson sees the role of the nurse as helping patients to reach independence, to give love and support when they feel ill but to help them take responsibility for their own planned care. In this country we have until very recently tended to take control over patients as soon as they enter the ward. This is demonstrated, for example, in our requiring of them to wear night clothes as soon as they are admitted. We tell them what they can have, when and sometimes even where: 'You have your meals at the table not in bed.' Thus rather than encourage the adult state we encourage the patient to regress to the dependent child state. In an attempt to move away from this model of care many hospitals have introduced the nursing process (see Fig. 1.4). One of the central aims of this process is to help the nurse help patients to the state of independence through being responsible for the care they are to receive, setting realistic goals, admitting that they need help but prepared to do what they can for themselves and the NURSE LETTING THEM.

1.4   Meeting the safety needs of the patient

Before we sit back in comfort knowing that this is the care that we give, how many wards have you worked on where the patients are in charge of their own drug therapy? The nurse's role here is to check that patients have an adequate supply, help those patients remember to take them and teach patients all they need to know about the tablets, how to recognize dangerous side-effects and what to do should such effects occur. Most units take any drugs that the patients have on them away during the admission procedure. Before we totally decry this practice we must remember the safety needs of the patient. It can be dangerous to mix certain drugs or the prescribed drugs could be rendered ineffective if mixed with some that the patient has brought unknown to the staff from home. The staff and patient must work together if the

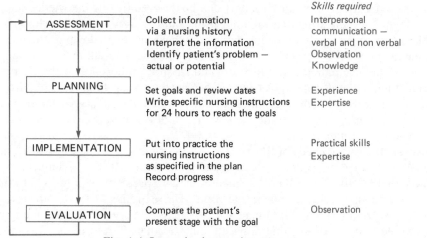

Fig. 1.4 Stages in the nursing process

patient is to be safe. However, when patients are discharged they are not going to have the nurses doing the drug round. Elderly people particularly are at risk of being confused over their drug administration. How much better it would be if we taught the patients while they were with us, for then we could keep a watchful eye and know when it would be safe for them to go home because they had demonstrated their ability to administer safely the drugs that they must continue to take.

Maslow (1954) formulated a positive theory of motivation derived from clinical experience which by integrating earlier theories arrives at a holistic–dynamic theory. He describes human beings as having a hierarchy of human needs which are as follows:

Basic physiological needs The need for the body to be in homeostasis; the need for air, food, water, warmth, etc.

Safety needs Security, stability, dependency, protection, freedom from fear, from anxiety, and from chaos, need for structure, laws, limits, etc.

Love, affection and belongingness needs – need to feel loved and wanted by others.

Esteem needs Need for self-respect or self-esteem and for the esteem of others.

Self-actualization Desire/need for self-fulfilment.

What Maslow meant by a hierarchy of needs is that we will not be aware of needs at the top end of the ladder if needs at the bottom end have not been fulfilled. For example, if a person is literally dying of hunger he is not going to be worrying about the promotional aspects of his work. This can be translated to our daily work on the wards. If a patient is in pain, there is no way that he is going to be able to look towards the goals of rehabilitation. Take the pain away or at least make it bearable and the patient will be able to take the first faltering steps towards, for example, the desired goal of mobility. Thus Maslow's hierarchy of needs (see Fig.1.5) may help us as nurses to help the patients to set realistic goals.

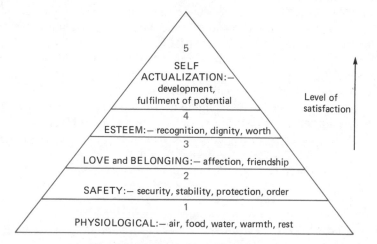

Fig. 1.5 Maslow's hierarchy of needs

One of the basic needs is safety. Safety can be ensured by our knowledge and observance of the code for fires, ensuring that the floor is dry, and preventing people slipping and falling. This will include reporting and dealing with safety hazards, even down to the use of cot sides. Such areas as our strict observance of an aseptic technique is essential – the patient came to be healed not to be given an added infection – and rigorous adherence to the hospital policy on drugs and their administration. As nurses we become very familiar with drugs and their administration, thus we can be tempted to cut corners. Accidents do happen. Patients are given the wrong drug or dose, sometimes with a fatal outcome. Should this occur the safety needs would not be met.

However, the safety needs of the patient must not be met at the expense of depriving the individual of his freedom, particularly his freedom of choice. It was Vivienne Wellburn (1980) who stated that, 'to live is to risk. . . . Prevention has a break-even point. Up to that point it is helpful, beyond that point it can be harmful.' The extreme of this conflict was brilliantly highlighted in Brian Clark's (1981) play *Whose Life is it Anyway?* Here a young man decides that his whole body is 'dead', that is paralysed, and that therefore his life-support machine should be switched off. The play is about the arguments for and against this course of action.

One of the basic needs for most individuals is to feel that they are in control. Some would argue that this is impossible but in a narrow sense we all like to think that we are in control, as can be seen by our preoccupation to plan ahead.   It is the feeling of no longer being in control that contributes to some people's fear of hospitals. They do not know what is going on or how to break into what at times must seem like a conspiracy of silence. Nurse says she does not know and to ask sister. Who is that? How will I recognize her? When is she on duty? Against this background patients do not know what to expect or how to prepare themselves, so often they end up thinking the worst and becoming extremely anxious. If we are to promote independence and the feeling of well-being then we must each play our part in ensuring that the patient is well informed. According to Hayward (1975) information is the prescription against pain. The most junior nurse can ensure that the patient knows the layout of the ward, the ward routine and who's who. You can explain each procedure in words the patient can understand and give time to ask questions, express fears or worries and state their preferences.

1.5   Nursing models

The ideas expressed so far in this chapter form the foundation of many nursing models. According to McGlynn (1983) a model is a

'representation of a structure, or the symbolic representation of an idealised situation, which shares the structure of the actual situation. It is a conceptual mirror, never reality.'

Thus a nursing model is a concept of what nursing is. Models are used as a tool to assess patient's needs/problems. There are many models of nursing but two you may know are Roper's Activities of Daily Living (1979) and Orem's Conceptual Model (Self-Care Deficit Model) (1980). Many schools of nursing have developed their own models.

In this unit we have briefly looked at the promotion of health through meeting the safety needs of the patient and ways of promoting independence and the feeling of well-being. As we have considered the three aspects of personality which can affect our reactions to situations, so we can consider three levels to our actions. As a baby we are totally dependent on our mother figure. What is sometimes referred to as the 'terrible twos' is that stage of toddlerhood where the child begins to seek for independence. Eventually as the child reaches maturity he begins to realize that an individual cannot stand alone. Then comes the stage of inter-dependence, the time of giving and receiving, of serving and being served, of loving and being loved. In the text so far we have talked only about dependence and independence, not because we do not recognize the stage or importance of interdependence, but because it is rarely the nurse's role in the acute situation to facilitate this aspect of life.

These aspects are summarized in the competences listed on page 1 which are required if the trained nurse is to fulfil the Code of Professional Conduct (page 147). Refer to your personal tutor, or use the books lists below, if you need clarification on any of the issues raised.

For a quick and easy revision test on this unit turn to page 109.

References

Berne, E., *Transactional Analysis in Psychotherapy* (Condor books, 1961)
Berne, E., *Games People Play: Psychology of Human Relationships* (Penguin, 1964)
Clark, B., *Whose Life is it Anyway?* (Amber Lane Productions, 1981)

Hayward, J., *Information – A Prescription against Pain* (RCN 1975)

Henderson, V., *Nature of Nursing* (Collier Macmillan, 1966)

Maslow, A. H., *Motivation and Personality* (Harper and Row, 1954)

McGlynn, J., 'The Unfolding of Ideas' (*Nursing Mirror,* January 12th 1983)

Villière, M. F., *Transactional Analysis at Work* (Prentice-Hall, 1981)

Welburn, V., *Postnatal Depression* (Manchester University Press, 1980)

World Health Organization, *Chronicle of the W.H.O.* (Annexe 1, vol 1, nos 1 to 12, W.H.O. Intrim Commission, New York)

Further reading

Boore, J. R. P., *Prescription for Recovery* (Churchill Livingstone, 1978)

Dubos, R., *The Mirage of Health* (Allen and Unwin Ltd, 1960)

Dunn, H. L., 'Positive Wellness in the Human National Posture' (Development note no 58, DAP 7, Washington D.C.)

Harris, T. A., *I'm O.K. – You're O.K.* (Pan books, 1973)

Orem, D., *Nursing Concepts of Practice* (McGraw Hill, 1980)

Roper, N., 'Nursing Based on Model of Living', in College, M. and Jones, D. (Eds) *Readings in Nursing* (Churchill Livingstone, 1979)

Roy, S.C., *Introduction to Nursing: An Adaptation Model* (Prentice-Hall Inc., 1976)

2 Care of the patient with problems in eating and drinking

2.1 Introduction

We all have our own body image, which is perceived by ourselves and others. Often these views do not coincide with reality and obesity and emaciation can be regarded as 'normal' by the individual. Therefore, when is a person over-weight or under-weight?

Standardized scales for height and weight for men and women have been compiled as a guideline only, and of course we all vary owing to genetic, social, economic and environmental factors. When body weight is a problem, these factors may need to be assessed, and advice given with continued support in the community.

Owing to physical and emotional distress weight may alter, and any sudden weight change should be investigated by medical staff. Often patients are assessed by the general practitioner or may be admitted to hospital for investigation of weight loss, or to reduce weight. This unit then will consider the problems of weight loss and weight gain.

2.2 Care of the patient with weight loss

Weight loss may be due to four main factors:

1 Loss of appetite, or inability to eat – unconscious patient.
2 Inability to absorb nutrients in the bowel – bowel disease.
3 Inability to utilize nutrients by the cells – diabetes mellitus.
4 Food intake may be adequate but insufficient to meet increased metabolism:
   thyrotoxicosis.
   multiple injuries.

In all these situations an assessment of the activity of eating and drinking is required according to the daily activity of each individual patient. This may involve recording all food eaten, and accurately recording body weight and stool/vomit chart daily. Scales used must be accurately maintained and patients weighed the same time each day, in similar clothing, on the same scales.

Activity

1 Weigh yourself on more than one type of scale in the same clothing, same day, same hour. Do your results vary?
2 Whose responsibility is it in your Health District to maintain accuracy of scales?

Promotion of eating a healthy diet is very important in nursing, but what is a healthy diet? At the present time much of the mass media, magazines, etc., fill their pages with ideas as to what we should eat – advice to eat more fibre, less saturated fats (mainly animal products) and to try and keep the fat in our diet to polyunsaturated fats (vegetable origin). Sugar and salt are considered bad for us. Health food shops abound with various products, many of them quite expensive. So what does the nurse have to consider when advising patients on what to eat? You must assess the individual person.

1 **Age** – are they likely to want to change their eating habits? The elderly may find their food the main enjoyment of life and cannot really see why they should change.

2 **Income** – suggesting foods which are too expensive will not help the families on low incomes. The nurse, in the absence of a dietician, should be aware of prices and varieties of foods which provide a similar nutritional need.

3 **Social factors** – who does the shopping? Are we advocating plenty of fresh fruit and vegetables for a person who is housebound, or has arthritis in hands and main joints making shopping difficult. Could a home help be available to ease the situation here.

Activity

Assess the patient you are caring for. It could be a patient:

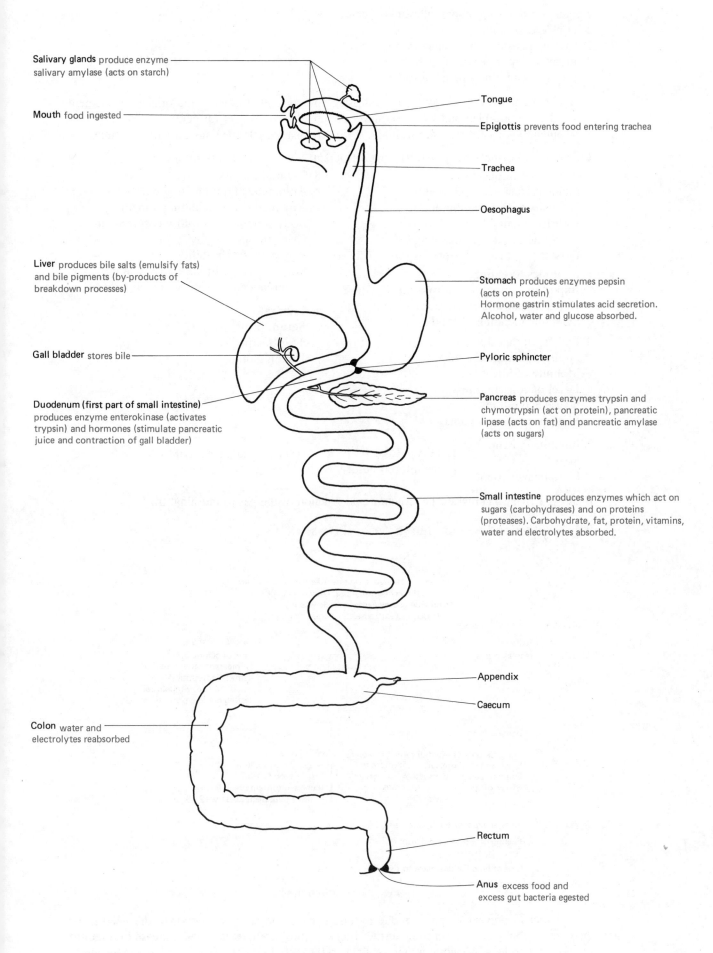

Salivary glands produce enzyme salivary amylase (acts on starch)

Mouth food ingested

Liver produces bile salts (emulsify fats) and bile pigments (by-products of breakdown processes)

Gall bladder stores bile

Duodenum (first part of small intestine) produces enzyme enterokinase (activates trypsin) and hormones (stimulate pancreatic juice and contraction of gall bladder)

Colon water and electrolytes reabsorbed

Tongue

Epiglottis prevents food entering trachea

Trachea

Oesophagus

Stomach produces enzymes pepsin (acts on protein) Hormone gastrin stimulates acid secretion. Alcohol, water and glucose absorbed.

Pyloric sphincter

Pancreas produces enzymes trypsin and chymotrypsin (act on protein), pancreatic lipase (acts on fat) and pancreatic amylase (acts on sugars)

Small intestine produces enzymes which act on sugars (carbohydrases) and on proteins (proteases). Carbohydrate, fat, protein, vitamins, water and electrolytes absorbed.

Appendix

Caecum

Rectum

Anus excess food and excess gut bacteria egested

Fig. 2.1 Structure and functions of the gastro-intestinal tract

1 ready for discharge home following surgery,
2 an elderly person,
3 a young person with a family to provide for,
4 an unemployed person, or
5 a person with a nutritional disorder.

Consider the items listed below when assessing your patient. Compare the original assessment sheet of your care plan and what you have identified as a result of furthering your assessment. Now amend your care plan accordingly, setting realistic goals for your patient to attain.

1 Details of normal eating pattern – age of person, details of dietary intake.

2 Any social implication:
  Financial factors implicated?
  Difficulty with obtaining food?
  Housing – stairs/lift?
  Shopping – walking? Carrying?
  Person responsible for preparation of food.

3 Attitudes to eating:
  Importance of eating/enjoyment of eating.
  Religious/cultural restrictions.
  Symbolic meaning of food.

4 Factors in digestion:
  Ability to swallow.
  Mobility of intestine.
  Level of consciousness.
  Nausea/vomiting.
  State of teeth and gums.

5 General factors:
  Any medication affecting emotional state.
  Any medication affecting appetite.
  Body weight, skin fold measurement.
  Grip strength.
  Any physical disability.
  Recent change in life pattern – e.g.
    bereavement, shift work, night duty.

6 Laboratory investigation:
  Serum proteins.
  Transferrin
  Haemoglobin.

7 Immune system:
  Skin tests.
  Lymphocyte count. } ability of the body to respond to substances it is likely to have encountered before.

Figure 2.1 (page 11) revises the structure and function of the gastro-intestinal tract.

2.3   Factors influencing nutrition in illness

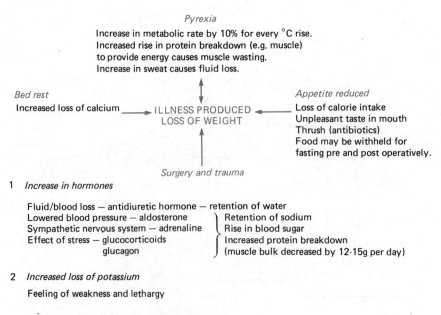

Fig. 2.2 Nutrition in illness

  In order to prevent weight loss due to illness, either physical or emotional, the need is for increased carbohydrates to prevent further breakdown of body tissues, and increased protein to replace protein loss. A calorie intake of 4000–5000 kcal (16.8–21 MJ) may be required per 24 hours to prevent weight loss in situations following major surgery, burns or trauma.

2.4 Nutrition of the patient unable to eat or drink

There are many reasons why patients are unable to eat or drink for varying periods, amongst which are reasons of reduced consciousness. Obviously, patients who are unconscious for longer than 36–48 hours will require nutritional intake in order to survive. Any patients who are obese or emaciated are at risk if their body is not provided with nutrients. The obese patient will need to reduce weight, but some carbohydrate is required to enable the fat stores to be utilized by the body completely, or ketoacidosis will occur. This state in turn decreases the level of consciousness, if ketone levels are high.

Ketoacidosis increases the risk of pressure sores because all body functions are reduced in an acidotic environment.

The emaciated patient is at risk from pressure sores if sufficient care is not provided to spread the pressure between the areas of pressure and the mattress (see the Norton scale in Section V). Decreased nutritional intake increases weight loss or breakdown (catabolism) of the body protein. The blood urea value will rise, especially if renal function is impaired. Elevated urea concentration in body tissues increases the breakdown of tissues and reduces the ability to heal. Nutrition, it can be seen, is vital if the patient is unable to eat or drink normally.

Activity

Assess the nutritional intake of patients in your existing area of care.

1 Patients requiring to be fasted:

> pre-post operatively,
> for special investigations,
> unconscious patients,
> pyrexial patients,
> patients with massive tissue destruction–burns/trauma,
> regeneration–skin conditions.

Consider particularly protein intake.

2 Study the RCN Research Project 'Nil by Mouth' (see page 19 for full reference).

There are two main routes through which the patient may be fed:

1 The enteral route
2 The parenteral route

The **enteral route** is the preferred route because it resembles normal eating and drinking. A fine-bore nasogastric tube is passed into the stomach, and its position needs to be assessed by X-ray. Problems may arise as a result of enteral feeding and these have been identified as follows (Hanson, 1975):

1 Abdominal cramps
2 Gastric distension
3 Diarrhoea
4 Nausea
5 Vomiting
6 Dehydration
7 Hypernatraemia (increased blood sodium levels)
8 Nasopharyngeal ulceration
9 Aspiration pneumonia

The patient must be carefully assessed prior to enteral feeding. Firstly it must be ascertained that the bowel is functioning normally. In some cases of unconsciousness and trauma, a paralytic ileus may develop, and therefore bowel sounds need to be present. The feed must be carefully chosen by the medical staff and the dietician. The age of the patient and body weight are important. Preparation of the feed is very important too because the patient is often in a severely debilitated state. Any bacterial infection from contaminated food would severely hinder the progress of the patient. The temperature of the feed, frequency of the feed, rate of giving the feed are important according to the ability to ingest and absorb the nutrients according to the individual needs of the patient.

Diarrhoea may be a problem of enteral feeding owing to the high concentration (osmolarity) of the feeds. Not only does the patient lose the fluid of the actual feed, but they are further dehydrated by the high osmolarity drawing liquid from the blood into the intestine. In order to prevent this, feeds are often diluted at the commencement of enteral feeding, and gradually increased in concentration so that the body becomes slowly adjusted to the full-strength feed.

The rate of giving of the feed is important; it may be given as bonus feeds throughout the 'normal waking hours', or given continuously as a 'drip' feed. Both methods have advantages in varying situations, but 'drip' feeding means the reservoir of food is suspended in a warm environment and the bacterial content is rapidly increased with up to 10 000 000 (10^7) organisms per ml feed.

Strict conditions of absolute cleanliness and sometimes sterile feeds are essential for the preparation of all ingredients in the diet to prevent gastroenteritis.

The **parenteral route** is an alternative route for feeding patients. The selection of patients for this method of providing nutrition should be carefully considered because of three reasons:

1 Danger of air embolism and perforation of blood vessel during insertion of subclavian line
2 Risk of septicaemia
3 Cost – very expensive

Insertion of the intravenous catheter is usually via the subclavian vein. This site is a 'short route' for the catheter tip into the great veins, and this enables dilution of the nutrients by a large volume of blood returning to the heart. This dilution lessens the risk of thrombo-phlebitis. Preferably, the catheter is inserted in the theatre or clinical room, under strict asepsis.

The patient is placed in a head-down position to increase the thoracic pressure and lessen the risk of air entering the catheter, producing an air embolus. The catheter site must be cleaned thoroughly, and the catheter is usually stitched in place. The area is occluded with a sealed dressing – e.g. OpSite. This dressing facilitates clear vision to monitor for any evidence of inflammation. The nurse should monitor the patient carefully for any circulatory collapse, or respiratory embarrassment after the catheter is inserted because the veins may be perforated during the procedure and a haemothorax or pneumothorax may be produced. The feeds are usually prepared by the pharmacy staff under sterile conditions, to ensure sterility of the feed. The container is sufficiently large to accommodate the full 24-hour feed to prevent bag changing in the ward. Preferably the giving set should be changed daily at the same time as the fresh feed is commenced, to reduce bacterial contamination. An accurate record must be maintained of the patient's temperature, pulse and fluid balance.

Activity

1 Look up your health district policy regarding the administration of parenteral nutrition, with regard to:
    (a) who may check feeds;   **(b)** change giving sets;   **(c)** change dressings;
    (d) precautions to be taken to prevent infection, and to assess whether infection has occurred.
2 Visit your pharmacist to identify the precautions taken in the sterile room when making additives to intravenous fluids. Examine ward practices. Can they be improved?

2.5   The role of the nurse in investigations of eating and drinking

Barium swallow/barium meal/follow-through

The preparation of patients for this investigation is simply fasting the patient prior to the X-ray. However, the patient is often very apprehensive about swallowing a large quantity of barium. The nurse's role is to lessen anxiety by discussing with the patient the following points:

1 Time of X-ray – need for fasting.
2 Barium can be flavoured – ascertain patient's preference.
3 If screening (barium swallow) is required, this takes place in a darkened room. Patients who are elderly may have difficulty with balance, etc. Well-fitting shoes may be required to ensure safety of patient. Warn the X-ray department if there is likely to be a problem with balance.
4 The patient will have pale stools after X-ray.
5 Barium is heavy and the patient will have a feeling of fullness, after swallowing substance.

6 Fear of vomiting and making a mess is an unspoken fear in most patients. Reassurance about nature of barium, etc may help relax the patient. Listen to his or her anxieties.

7 If a 'follow-through' is required, the patient must understand why there will be several visits to the X-ray department during the day. Normal eating and drinking are usually allowed after the initial X-ray.

Jejunal biopsy

This procedure requires the swallowing of a Crosby capsule which is attached to a fine-bore plastic tube, and it passes into the jejunum by the peristaltic action of the gastro-intestinal tract. The capsule has within it a blade, which can be triggered by applying suction at the end of the tube with a syringe. The capsule and tube are then withdrawn (see Fig. 2.3). Swallowing the capsule is the greatest problem for the patient, and anxiety is created by fear of vomiting. Anxiety needs to be lessened by explaining the advantages of obtaining tissue by this method:

1 It is quick – does not require an operation.   **3** It is painless.

2 It is safer than surgery.   **4** Preparation is fasting.

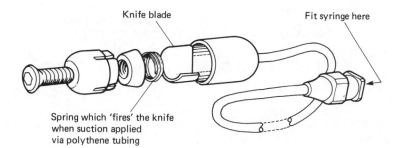

Knife blade   Fit syringe here

Spring which 'fires' the knife when suction applied via polythene tubing

Fig. 2.3 The Watson intestinal biopsy capsule

The capsule is approximately the size of the top of a small finger, and to swallow it is similar to swallowing a small bolus of food. Instruct the patient when to relax by breathing gently through the mouth. If the capsule is cooled slightly it sometimes is felt to be more acceptable. The distance from the mouth to the stomach can be roughly ascertained by marking the plastic tube. Place the patient in the lateral position after the tube has been passed. As the capsule moves into the duodenum and jejunum its position is checked by X-ray. After the biopsy has been taken, the patient should be observed for any evidence of abdominal pain or discomfort, rise in pulse, or fall in blood pressure which may be evident if bleeding or perforation of the bowel occurs. Food and drink may be taken normally after the biopsy is obtained.

Oesophagoscopy/Gastroscopy

This examination entails passing a fibre-optic tube into the stomach, duodenum or common bile duct according to the area of vision required. The advantages of this procedure should be given to the patient, because most patients are very apprehensive of any examination of the stomach. The patient requires preparation as for an anaesthetic with a pre-medication usually given. Often the patient does not remember the actual procedure because a small dose of intra-venous diazepam may be given prior to the endoscopy if the patient is very apprehensive. The throat is sprayed with a local anaesthetic to reduce the gag reflex and the tube quickly passed down the oesophagus to the required level. Any biopsy, photograph or calculi may be retrieved, or dye can be injected as far as the common bile duct to assess patency.

After the patient returns to the ward, oral fluids should be withheld until considered safe by the medical staff because of reduced cough and swallow reflex or possible risk of haemorrhage. The patient needs to rest. If seen as a day case he/she should not drive a car but arrangements should be made for him/her to be accompanied home.

Activity

Give four suspected diagnoses in which the above investigations may be required.

(see Fig. 2.4)

2.6 The problem of malabsorption from the gastro-intestinal tract (see Fig. 2.4)

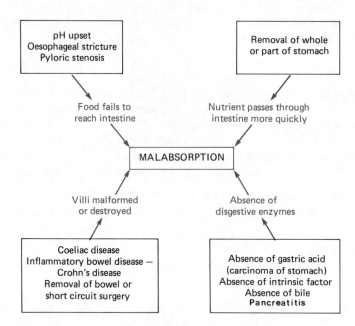

Fig. 2.4 Malabsorption

The nursing care of patients with malabsorption syndrome will initially require a careful medical and nursing assessment regarding:

1 Previous medical history
2 Evidence of pain, indigestion, vomiting, diarrhoea
3 Details of vomit–frequency (before/during/after meals)
4 Amount
5 Colour

6 Details of pain:
  Day, night or both
  Before meals
  During meals
  After meals
  Any particular foods
  On lying down
7 Type of pain:
  Gnawing
  Colicky/spasms
  Localized, generalized

8 Diarrhoea:
  Frequency
  Approximate volume
  Colour–blood stained, mucus, dark, pale putty
  Odour–normal/offensive
  Stools sink in the pan or float?
  Explosive–gas present
  Fatty in consistency
  Containing undigested food

Patients with a problem of malabsorption are not only emaciated, but anaemia often accompanies the condition. This may be due to chronic inflammation causing chronic blood loss from the bowel, loss of intrinsic factor, or failure to absorb iron or vitamin B_{12}. Anaemia and lack of nutrients to the body produce problems of lethargy, weakness, breathlessness on exertion, and therefore, the promotion of rest and sleep is very important. Because of the nature of the condition, rest and sleep are often disturbed, and anxiety levels are increased, creating a vicious circle. The nurse should realize that rest does not necessarily mean no activity. A patient normally quite active will resent being confined to bed completely except for toilet purposes. This increases frustration and anxiety. Reading or some form of work suitable to facilitate physical rest may even be beneficial. Often a compromise may be made between the opposing needs. If anxiety is reduced the gastro-intestinal tract may function more effectively. Diazepam in small doses may be prescribed to assist relaxation.

Smoking should be discouraged for patients with gastro-intestinal tract problems. It has been well demonstrated that smoking has the following effects on the body:

1 Reduces vitamin C levels in the blood – reduced ability to heal.
2 Causes vasoconstriction – less blood supply to tissues.
3 Reduces oxygen levels in blood – reduced ability to heal.
4 Smoke enters the stomach and can cause irritation of the mucosa.
5 Reduces senses of taste and smell.   6 Reduces appetite.

Patients who smoke heavily, especially if they are tired and anxious, find that to stop smoking is very difficult. The reason for reducing smoking and the benefits to the patient should be discussed with the patient. Often medication or contact through the organization ASH may assist the patient. Nurses too should remember that if they smoke, it can be detected on the breath and clothes, which may increase a patient's desire to smoke. If patients are encouraged to set their own targets to reduce smoking, e.g. set a daily allowance, they may actually smoke less than patients **told** not to smoke, who have a cigarette frequently in the toilet! Care and understanding should help to develop a greater commitment by the patient. Praise for achievement, rather than rebuke or reprimand for failure, is much more effective.

Care plan for a patient with malabsorption problems

Problem	Aim of care	Nursing care
Weight loss	Assessment of appetite Assessment of weight loss To prevent further weight loss and promote weight gain	Detail of actual dietary intake/vomiting, etc. Weigh daily – same time of day, similar clothing. Measure skin fold thickness. Administer dietary intake according to medical and nursing assessment: parenteral nutrition; enteral nutrition; dietary supplement.
Tiredness and lethargy	Promote rest and prevent complications of bed rest Correct any anaemia	Ensure good night's sleep and rest periods during the day. Aids to promote comfort and prevent pressure sores – assess Norton Scale (see Appendix). Change position 2 hourly. Monitor skin for redness. Exercise legs. Deep breathing. Full blood count. Group cross match blood. Care of blood transfusion if necessary.

Altered stool and pattern of elimination	Monitor stool pattern to evaluate treatment	Stool chart: Frequency
		(see Appendix) Consistency } Stools
		                         Colour/Odour
		Specimen for bacteriology
		                         parasitology
		                         fat content
		                         occult blood

Patient very susceptible to infection	Promote personal hygiene of patient and ensure all staff are instructed in preventing spread of infection and cleaning methods	Keep the patient's skin clean, dry and supple. Prevent any cracking of dry skin. Protect skin from excoriation. Provide hand washing facility after elimination. Parenteral line – implement district policy concerning prevention of infection.
Anxiety about condition or occupation, etc	Keep patient fully informed and assess patient's needs regularly by promoting discussion	Inform and discuss fully all investigations. Discuss the treatment and any implications of the treatment. Discuss care plan with the patient. Medical staff should see patient regularly and discuss care.

2.7 The problem of obesity

Obesity is usually due to over-eating and lack of exercise, although there are people who eat very few calories, take exercise and yet do not lose weight. These people are in the minority.

   Obesity is regarded as being detrimental to most body systems, and therefore prevention of obesity or its reduction are advocated. In some health districts applicants for nurse training have been refused entry if they are considered overweight for their height. They may re-apply if they lose weight. Our diet is usually at fault. We are what we eat! Foods high in carbohydrate and fats – chips, bread and butter, ice-cream, wine, beer and sweets to name but a few – are often eaten in excess. Advertising has a devastating effect upon what we eat.

Activity

Monitor the food/drink advertisements – what foods do they advertise? Are they high in sugars (carbohydrates) and fats?

The general public is gradually becoming more aware of the need for fibre in the diet. This is important because much bowel disorder is considered to be due to a lack of fibre. Bulky fibre increases peristalsis of the bowel by increasing stretch and contraction of the muscle fibres. Transit time through the bowel is reduced. Sugar and fats in the diet have also been found to have lower rates of absorption, and blood sugar levels are evened out, instead of peaks of high blood sugar after meals. This factor is important because it means that if the sugar is utilized evenly by the body, less is available for deposition as fat. The diabetic patient can benefit from this effect of fibre and most dieticians advocate a high-fibre diet.

Cream, butter, margarine, oil, oily fish, eggs and fat meat are all high-risk sources of fat and, therefore, any person wanting to reduce weight should remove or reduce these substances. The animal fats are considered to increase atheroma formation in the arteries, and polyunsaturated fats – e.g. vegetable oils – reduce the risk. It should be remembered, however, that any form of fat is a rich source of calories, and if weight is to be reduced, all fat must be reduced to a minimum (see tables in Appendix).

Activity

How many calories are yielded by 1 g of carbohydrate, protein and fat?

The effects of obesity upon the body systems

1 Reduced ability to be active. Breathlessness becomes a problem more quickly when an obese person is active. This is because the body has an increased oxygen demand due to skeletal muscle needing more oxygen and producing more carbon dioxide. When moving, the heart rate increases and the respirations increase to supply the body tissues with oxygen and remove the waste carbon dioxide. If the arteries contain deposits of atheroma, the blood supply to the muscles – especially the heart muscle – is reduced and angina may result. Fat too may be deposited around the heart and this also embarrasses the heart's action.

2 The abdominal wall and omentum are the main areas for storage of fat, but if this fat is excessive the diaphragm is unable to descend and the ribs cannot move upwards and outwards.

3 The skeletal system has to take more weight hanging on it, rather like an overloaded coathanger. Moving surfaces, e.g. joints, especially the hip and the knees which take the body weight, are affected. Any person suffering from osteoarthritis who has limited movement should be urged to lose weight if obesity is a problem. There is a greater risk of back injury in obese people and this is of particular concern to nurses. They must get close to people when lifting or manoeuvrability may be hindered, increasing strain upon the lumbar spine.

4 The pancreas produces insulin to keep blood sugar levels within normal limits. If ingestion of carbohydrate is increased over a long period of time the production of insulin may be impaired by 'wearing out' of the gland. Often the mature-onset diabetic patient is overweight, though not always. Much research is being undertaken to identify causes of diabetes, which is on the increase in Western civilizations, together with obesity.

5 Haemorrhoids and varicose veins may be aggravated by obesity. Fat within the abdomen can cause pressure on veins, so reducing venous return. Reduced exercise because of obesity reduces the effect of the muscle pump in the legs and increases stasis of blood. Varicose veins and deep vein thrombosis may occur. High-carbohydrate, low-fibre diet also increases the tendency to constipation. Straining at stool increases the problems of haemorrhoids, and a full rectum of faeces increases the risk of varicose veins. Leg ulceration may develop as a result of poor venous return.

From this brief examination of the problems that obesity brings, you should see why encouraging patients to lose weight is important.

If anyone wishes to lose weight it should be reduced gradually, and be carefully controlled.

Medical advice may be necessary as 'crash diets' are often dangerous. The effect of group competition as in Weight Watchers is often an effective method of losing weight, but joining these groups is not free of charge. Proprietary slimming foods are expensive and medical advice should be sought, especially if excessive weight loss is required.

Emotional support and encouragement is very important. Often obesity is a problem within families and is mistaken as being hereditary. If a nutritional assessment is made, the diet of the family is often found to be at fault. Members of a family, e.g. husband and wife, can support each other when losing weight (see Fig. 2.5). Eating for comfort is a recognized phenomenon, and emotional problems may cause obesity. When some people are depressed or anxious they may over-eat, or lose their appetites. Obesity itself can increase depression, and a vicious circle ensues.

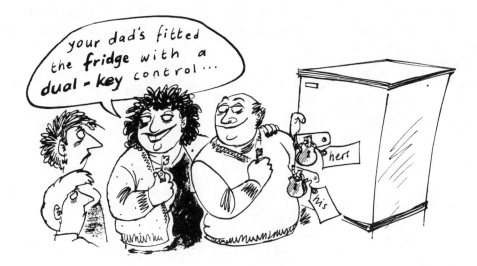

Fig. 2.5

For a quick and easy revision test on this unit turn to page 110.

Further reading

Beck, M. E., *Nutrition and Dietetics for Nurses* (Churchill Livingstone, 1972)

Brunner, L. S. and Suddarth, D. S., *Lippencott Manual of Nursing Practice* (Lippencott Nursing, 1982)

Clark, J. and James, E. (editors), 'Nutrition and Health' (*Nursing*, 1st series, no 11, all articles, March 1980)

Clark, J. and James, E. (editors), 'Nutrition in Illness' (*Nursing*, 1st series, no 12, all articles, April 1980)

Hamilton-Smith, S., *Nil by Mouth* (Royal College of Nursing, 1972)

James, E. H. and Dickerson, J. W. (editors), 'Nutrition' (*Nursing*, volume 2, nos 4 and 5, all articles, August and September 1982)

Nursing Mirror Supplement, 'Forum on Healthy Eating' (*Nursing Mirror*, July 12th 1979)

Rossiter, J. E., 'Problems of Dietary Change' (*Nursing* 2, vol 2, June 1982)

Shafer, K. N., Sawyer, J. R. *et al.*, *Medical-Surgical Nursing* International Student Edition (C. V. Mosby Co, 1979)

3 Care of the patient with fluid imbalance

3.1 The control of normal body fluid balance

Body fluids are normally maintained in balance between fluid loss and fluid intake: **homeostasis**.

The organs concerned with fluid loss are:

The kidneys – as urine.   The lungs   – as water vapour.
The skin   – as sweat.   The bowels – faeces.

60% – 70% of body weight is water in adults (see Fig. 3.1). Fluid is divided into three main body compartments, but fluid is constantly moving between these compartments, and there are forces controlling its exchange.

The body fluids are divided between:

1 The cells (intracellular compartment)	= 30 litres
2 The extracellular compartment	= 12 litres
3 The blood (in plasma)	= 3 litres
	= 45 litres

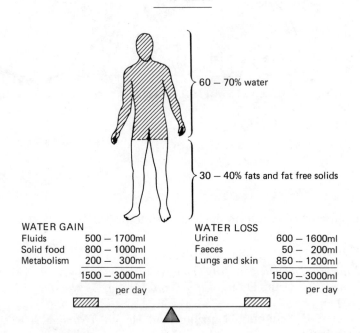

Fig. 3.1 Composition of the body and homeostasis

The patient with fluid imbalance has suffered upset to the balance between these compartments. When fluid is lost from the body it is the blood volume which is first depleted. This is then restored by fluid from the extracellular compartment and then finally from the cells (see Fig. 3.2).

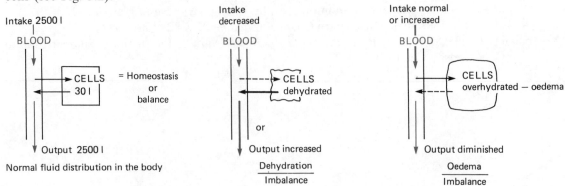

Fig. 3.2 Dehydration and oedema

The kidney is the main organ for regulation of fluid balance. Fig. 3.3 revises the structure and functions of the nephron.

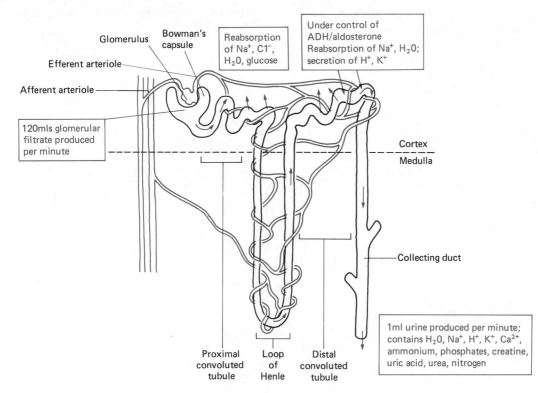

Fig. 3.3 Structure and functions of the nephron

Antidiuretic hormone (ADH) production is controlled by the posterior lobe of the pituitary gland. It detects over-concentrated blood reaching the brain and causes ADH to be released. ADH in turn stimulates thirst and reabsorption of more water in the kidney tubules. Diluted blood has the opposite effect of causing the pituitary to inhibit ADH production so causing sweating and increased water excretion.

Effect of environmental factors on fluid balance

Exercise and the environmental temperature affect fluid balance as shown in Fig. 3.4.

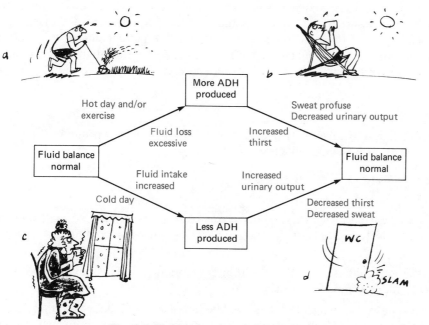

Fig. 3.4 Fluid balance and the environment

The effect of blood pressure on fluid balance

Activity

State briefly what you understand by osmosis and diffusion. How is the control of body fluids normally maintained?

Movement of fluid occurs across the blood capillary wall. Two main forces are responsible for homeostasis of body fluid (see Fig. 3.5):

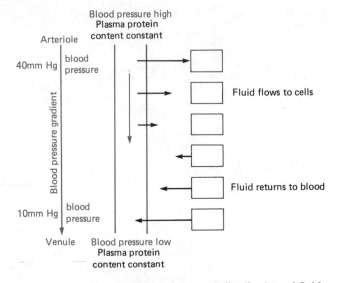

Fig. 3.5 Factors maintaining normal distribution of fluid between blood and tissues

1 Blood pressure gradient between arterioles and venules.
2 Osmotic pressure of the plasma proteins.

Plasma proteins, red cells and platelets normally stay within the blood vessels as they are too large to pass between the cells of the capillary wall. However, it is the plasma proteins (mainly plasma albumin) that exerts a pull (osmotic pressure) drawing water towards the capillary by osmosis. This force is normally constant. The blood pressure gradually falls the further the distance away from the heart. In the arteriole blood pressure is higher than in the venule.

In the arteriole the blood pressure exceeds the osmotic pressure of the plasma proteins, therefore the blood pressure forces fluid out to the cells taking dissolved substances with it, e.g. nutrients and electrolytes.

In the venule the osmotic pressure exceeds the blood pressure therefore pressure draws fluid back to the blood bringing with it waste products.

So we see that fluid balance depends not only on the balance of fluid intake and output, but also on the blood pressure in the capillaries and the osmotic pressure of the plasma proteins.

The shocked patient (lowered blood pressure) and the patient unable to obtain protein (poor diet), absorb protein (malabsorption) or manufacture protein (liver failure) may therefore suffer from oedema. For the effects of shock on fluid balance see Fig. 5.1 on page 51.

Activity

Revise the functions of the liver with respect to production of plasma proteins. What problems will reduced levels of protein production cause?

Principles of electrolyte balance and acid–base balance

Electrolyte balance

Electrolytes are substances which in solution can carry an electrical charge. This is because they contain positively and negatively charged particles which can combine to form a salt, as follows:

Sodium (Na^+) and chloride (Cl^-) make sodium chloride ($NaCl$–common salt). Potassium (K^+) and chloride (Cl^-) make potassium chloride (KCl).

These are substances with which the nurse will be familiar. The kidney maintains the balance of sodium by the action of **aldosterone** produced in the adrenal cortex, which regulates the reabsorption of sodium from the nephron. As sodium is reabsorbed by the body, acids and potassium are exchanged for the sodium. When diuretics are prescribed, they reduce the reabsorption of sodium by either antagonizing aldosterone or influencing the nephron itself. Care must be taken to ensure that the patient does not become depleted in potassium because of the resulting increased urinary output. Potassium is vital for the body cells to function. Effects of hypokalaemia (potassium depletion) are:

1 Tiredness   4 Abnormal heart rhythms   7 Death
2 Lethargy   5 Nausea/paralytic ileus
3 Faintness   6 Muscle weakness/cramps

Acid–base balance

Acids (H^+ ions) are ingested in the diet, and are produced too by the body as a result of metabolism. It is important that the body pH (acidity and alkalinity) remains constant.

The kidney excretes acids – hence urine is acid, and the kidney is also able to conserve bicarbonate (base) to neutralize acids. If the body becomes too acid (acidosis) or alkaline (alkalosis) then the cells cannot function and death could result.

To summarize – the main function of the kidney is to maintain homeostasis of (1) fluid balance; (2) electrolyte balance; (3) acid–base balance.

All of these functions are interrelated and often cannot be separated when considering disturbance of fluid balance.

In order to assess a patient's state of fluid balance the nurse must observe the total patient, including his or her behaviour. Knowledge of how fluid balance is maintained or factors that cause disturbance of balance is essential – e.g. shock and its causes, liver failure, renal failure, vomiting, diarrhoea, burns. Assessment includes monitoring accurately all intake and output of fluid and the effects upon the patient, especially the cardiovascular and respiratory systems.

Assessment of fluid balance

How do you assess fluid balance? A laborious way is to measure intake and output of fluid which is considered to be often inaccurate. This method does not measure all liquid in food, or fluid loss through sweat and faeces, etc. A more accurate measurement, if carried out properly, is to measure body weight. The person must be weighed accurately, at the **same time** of day, in the **same clothes** on the **same scales** which must be **accurately maintained**. When overall fluid gain or loss is the main consideration, and the patient is mobile, body weight is a more accurate measurement than a fluid balance chart. However, many patients require a more detailed assessment of body fluids, and therefore a chart facilitates divisions of intake and output. A fluid balance chart is in the Appendix.

3.2 Care of the patient with fluid loss

Fig. 3.6 illustrates the causes and symptoms of dehydration.

3.3 Care of the vomiting patient – intestinal obstruction (See Fig. 3.7)

Feeling nauseated and actually vomiting is a particularly distressing feature of being 'unwell'. There are many causes of vomiting.

Activity

See how many causes of vomiting you can list. To assist you, consider them under the following headings:

1 Dietary intake –
   Identify organisms, nature of spread.
   Substances causing allergy, poisons.
2 Drugs – identify groups of drugs.
3 Mechanical causes of disturbance in gastro-intestinal tract.
4 Inflammatory causes of disturbance in gastro-intestinal tract.
5 Neurological causes of vomiting.
6 Disorders of the renal tract.
7 Disorders of the liver.
8 Emotional disturbance.
9 Disorders of the endocrine system.

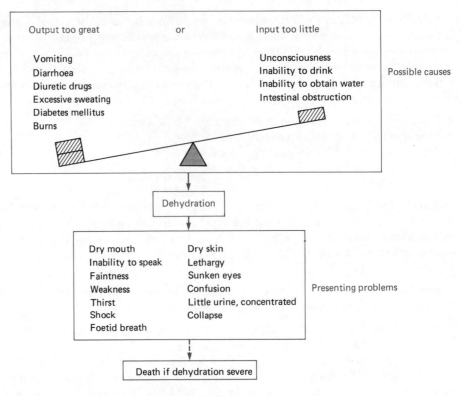

Fig. 3.6 Dehydration

Pain is a feature in many of the illnesses you have identified, whether it is headache, abdominal pain, pelvic pain, or any other pain, and of course vomiting may be the result of severe pain. Whatever the problem, vomiting will intensify pain due to the increase in intracranial pressure, intrathoracic pressure and abdominal and pelvic pressures. To alleviate vomiting is therefore important.

Nursing measures to alleviate vomiting

1 Avoid smell related to food or body odours if the patient is nauseated:

Consider the patient's environment.
Consider the patient's own situation – vomit bowl; tissues; clothing (odorous excreta, including sweat).

2 Keep the mouth fresh and clean:

Mouthwashes.
Clean teeth with toothbrush if patient is conscious because a dry mouth causes crusting of saliva.

3 Obtain a nursing assessment of vomiting by ascertaining:
   (a) Any evidence of pain? Location, description, time related to food, how long has it existed?
   (b) Type of food – especially if food poisoning suspected.
   (c) Nature of vomit – undigested food, bile stained, coffee grounds (haematemesis), faecal fluid.
   (d) Volume: Assess general appearance for evidence of dehydration.
               Tongue/mouth – dry/moist/furred tongue/bleeding gums.
               Breath – acetone smell/respiration rate increased?
               Monitor blood pressure/pulse rate for shock.
               Measure specific gravity of urine and ketones.
               Measure volume of urine/vomit.
   4 Depending upon the degree of illness, the patient's weight may be required.

These observations should be recorded in the nursing report.

Activity

List the complications of an infected mouth. Examine research on methods to clean mouth. How does this relate to nursing practice?

Remember that to vomit is **not normal**.

Vomiting means **loss of fluid**, also gastric acid, vital vitamins, nutrients and electrolytes either in undigested form or because of the loss of desire to eat and drink.

Vomit may **obstruct the airway**.

Medical measures to alleviate vomiting

1 Pass a nasogastric tube. This has two main functions: it keeps the stomach empty of fluid (therefore minimizes the fluids passing to the intestine); and it minimizes vomiting and pain.

2 If the nasogastric tube is left on free drainage it enables gas to pass up the tube, and therefore assists in relieving abdominal distension, and related pain. Remember to advise your patient of the **advantages** of having the tube passed as this will help him or her to accept this unpleasant procedure to be undertaken.

3 Administration of anti-emetic drugs.

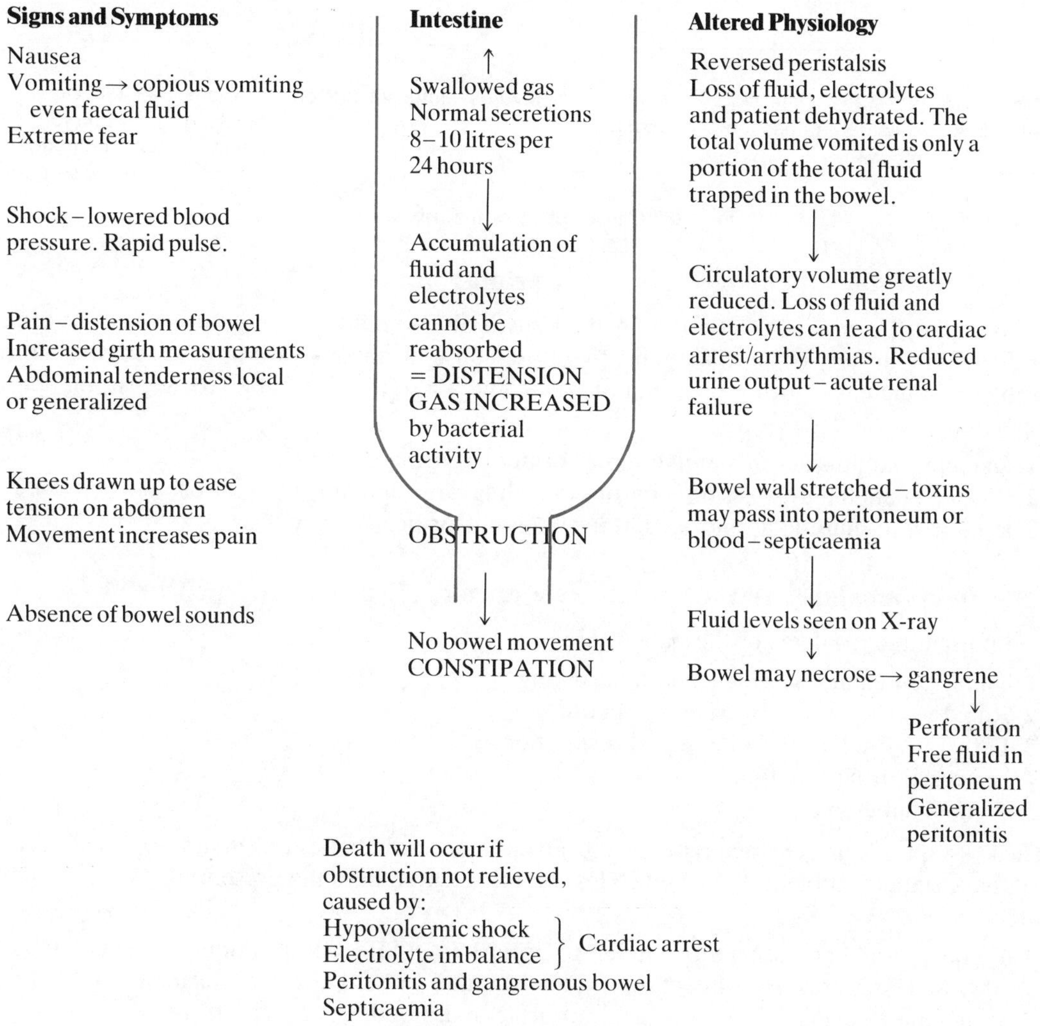

Signs and Symptoms	**Intestine**	**Altered Physiology**
Nausea	↑	Reversed peristalsis
Vomiting → copious vomiting even faecal fluid	Swallowed gas	Loss of fluid, electrolytes and patient dehydrated. The
Extreme fear	Normal secretions 8–10 litres per 24 hours	total volume vomited is only a portion of the total fluid trapped in the bowel.
	↓	
Shock – lowered blood pressure. Rapid pulse.	Accumulation of fluid and	Circulatory volume greatly reduced. Loss of fluid and
	electrolytes cannot be	electrolytes can lead to cardiac arrest/arrhythmias. Reduced
Pain – distension of bowel	reabsorbed	urine output – acute renal
Increased girth measurements	= DISTENSION	failure
Abdominal tenderness local or generalized	GAS INCREASED by bacterial activity	
		Bowel wall stretched – toxins
Knees drawn up to ease tension on abdomen		may pass into peritoneum or blood – septicaemia
Movement increases pain	OBSTRUCTION	
	↓	Fluid levels seen on X-ray
Absence of bowel sounds	No bowel movement	↓
	CONSTIPATION	Bowel may necrose → gangrene
		↓
		Perforation Free fluid in peritoneum Generalized peritonitis

Death will occur if
obstruction not relieved,
caused by:
Hypovolcemic shock ⎫
Electrolyte imbalance ⎬ Cardiac arrest
Peritonitis and gangrenous bowel ⎭
Septicaemia

Fig. 3.7 Diagram to illustrate how the altered physiology of intestinal obstruction produces the associated signs and symptoms.

Activity

Look up the names of anti-emetic drugs, their action, and possible side-effects.

The patient becomes severely dehydrated and will require urgent replacement of fluids. There are disorders that produce vomiting, but in which the degree of dehydration appears in excess of the severity of vomiting, e.g. lower intestinal obstruction. Any disorder causing dehydration is a potentially life-threatening situation because of fluid imbalance. Remember – the cells of the body eventually lose fluid and vital potassium from within their walls, which slows down their ability to function. This includes the heart muscle, therefore severe dehydration can produce abnormal heart rhythms, the bowel will reduce peristaltic action and severe behavioural disorders including coma can occur.

Activity

Produce a care plan for a patient with intestinal obstruction, prior to going to theatre.

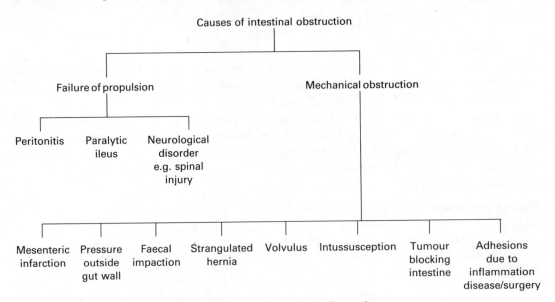

Fig. 3.8 Causes of intestinal obstruction

3.4 Care of the patient with increased urinary output

It has already been stated that normally the body is able to regulate fluid output by increasing or decreasing urinary output. We must therefore consider nursing care in illnesses where the problem is increased urinary output because the kidney is not able to adjust the fine regulations as in:

1 Diabetes mellitus and hyperglycaemia (osmotic diuresis).
2 Chronic renal failure – loss of nephrons excreting large amounts of urea (osmotic diuresis).
3 Lack of anti-diuretic hormone – pituitary tumour or head injury.

3.5 Fluid imbalance in the patient with uncontrolled diabetes mellitus

The presenting problems of the patient are:

1 Thirst that cannot be quenched by drinking.
2 Rapid weight loss despite good appetite.
3 Lethargy, tiredness and increased respiration.
4 Increased urinary output.
5 Abdominal cramp.

These symptoms are characteristic of the juvenile-onset diabetic; the mature-onset diabetic will have similar problems but of much less severity. Often here the presenting problems may be:

1 Frequent scalding on micturition due to urinary tract infection promoted by glycosuria.
2 May be respiratory tract infection ⎱ patient found to be diabetic on examination
3 Gangrene of digits ⎰ of urine and blood.

Why does a raised blood sugar increase the urinary output? First we need to consider the normal pathway of carbohydrates in our diet, very simply. Refer to Fig. 2.1 in Unit 2 to revise the digestion and absorption of carbohydrates.

In the kidney the sugar is normally all reabsorbed from the glomerular filtrate in the proximal tubule of the nephron. In diabetes the amount of sugar is too great for total reabsorption and the high osmolarity of filtrate inhibits reabsorption of water back into the blood, causing raised urinary output, **glycosuria**, **dehydration** and increased thirst.

In order to correct dehydration the principles of medical treatment are:

1 Infuse large volumes of fluids if dehydration is severe.
2 Administer insulin to reduce high blood sugar levels.

This treatment will reduce urinary output, to enable the patient to retain infused fluid. Nursing evaluation includes monitoring hourly urine totals, also monitoring the pulse rate, blood pressure and CVP. Report any abnormal rise immediately.

Severe electrolyte imbalance will have been created by increased urinary output and potassium loss. Treatment is therefore to replace potassium via an intravenous infusion according to the plasma electrolyte levels.

The patient will be acidotic (ketoacidosis) because in order to obtain energy the patient will have been using 'fat stores'. Fat cannot be completely metabolized in the absence of sugars (in this case sugar cannot be utilized) and ketones are the result of incomplete fat breakdown. Ketones should be reduced by the administration of insulin (see Fig. 3.9). Fig. 3.9 illustrates the causes of ketoacidosis.

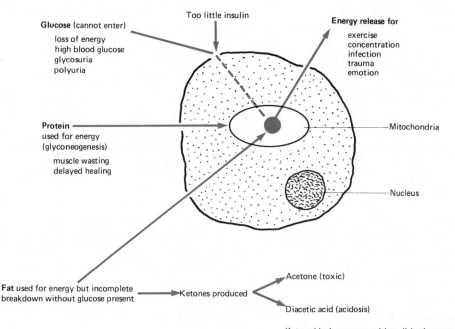

Fig. 3.9 Ketoacidosis

Care plan for a patient with diabetes mellitus in diabetic ketoacidosis and fluid imbalance

Problem	Aim	Nursing care
Patient drowsy/unconscious	Maintain vital body systems and prevent deterioration in condition	Lateral position – suction oxygen. Eye care two hourly. Change position two hourly. Support all limbs. Monitor pulse and blood pressure.
Excessive thirst and increased urinary output, weight loss	Restore normal body fluids Reduce urinary output Correct high blood sugar to within normal limits	Care of IV infusion (CVP). Monitor urinary output (hourly urine totals). Four hourly catheter care – catheter with 'sampling port'. Test urine for ward testing. Oral hygiene two hourly. Insulin IV/IM as prescribed. Monitor blood sugar levels.
Patient's skin hot and dry	Reduce body temperature by not more than 1°C	Fan, tepid sponging, cotton night-clothes. Assess susceptibility to pressure sores – Norton Scale.
Abdominal pain and cramps Nausea and vomiting	Prevent paralytic ileus	Assess for bowel sounds. If absent: pass nasogastric tube; aspirate hourly; leave on free drainage; withhold oral fluids.

When the condition improves an ongoing care plan is needed. This includes an educational programme for the new diabetic patient, and restabilization for the known diabetic, according to individual need.

A full nursing history will be taken to identify the cause of imbalance, and establish any emotional or social factors that may have contributed to the patient's condition.

Ongoing care must include a programme for the 'new diabetic' to understand his/her condition and promote health.

1 How would *you* teach the patient what diabetes is?
2 The need for treatment – the advantages being stressed so that a normal life can be achieved.

3 According to intellect of patient, design a programme that aims to achieve the following:
   (a) Understanding of dietary programme
   (b) Understanding of calculation of dosage of insulin and its safe administration
   (c) Ability to recognize hypoglycaemia and hyperglycaemia
   (d) Correct action to take in the event of being ill
   (e) Prevention of complications of diabetes by ensuring care of the feet and eyes and promotion of dietary fibre. Monitor 'normal' body weight. Understand the harmful effects of smoking – (page 17).
   (f) Safe care of the syringe, needles, etc and prevention of complications when administering insulin injections
   (g) Who to contact if help and advice is required
   (h) Understanding the need for continued medical support especially during adolescence, pregnancy, change in life pattern, change of job, and times of any emotional upset

3.6   Care of the patient with chronic renal failure

The patient with chronic renal failure has a progressive condition producing gradual destruction of the nephrons. There are many causes of renal failure as shown in Fig. 3.10. All of these causes of chronic renal failure may lead, through kidney damage, to hypertension, which then further damages the kidney. (Inappropriate renin production.)

Because of damaged nephrons the body is unable to excrete body waste and therefore harmful substances rise in the blood:

Urea from protein breakdown
Acids from the diet and body metabolism (metabolic acidosis)
Electrolyte imbalance due to loss of nephrons

The remaining nephrons endeavour to get rid of these substances and the filtrate contains a high concentration of urea. The urea has an osmotic effect in the filtrate and therefore inhibits the reabsorption of water. The patient with chronic renal failure is therefore unable to concentrate his urine even if the body is dehydrated.

Only in the terminal state will the urinary output decrease in volume. Metabolic acidosis will increase the respiratory rate, so more fluid will be lost through respiration.

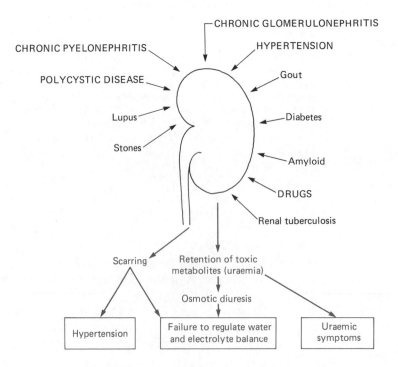

Fig. 3.10 Chronic renal failure

Urea will cause irritation of all of the body tissues:

1 The gastro-intestinal tract – diarrhoea, nausea and vomiting
2 The skin – urea frost from sweat – itching skin
3 The brain and nervous system – altered behaviour, altered consciousness and cramps
4 The body generally – weight loss due to reduced ability to absorb nutrients and anorexia, and dehydration causing marked debility

The kidney has an important function of producing hormones:

1 Renin – regulates blood pressure. In chronic renal failure, hypertension may be a problem causing headaches.
2 Erythropoietin – essential for red cell formation. In chronic renal failure, anaemia may exist, increasing tiredness and breathlessness.

Both of these states can produce left ventricular failure which increases problems of fluid imbalance in the lungs, producing breathlessness and poor cardiac output. Angina may result. These patients are usually aware of their progressive illness and both patients and relatives require constant support, by encouraging them to express their feelings and anxieties. The social worker, general practitioner and district nurse may all be involved in the patient's care, and therefore should be informed of any changes in treatment or condition prior to the patient's return to the community.

Care plan for patient with fluid imbalance due to chronic renal failure

Patient problem	Aim	Nursing care
Altered behaviour confusion/drowsiness	Ensure patient's safety Reduce toxic wastes in the body	Low bed. Cot sides as appropriate. Ensure continuity of care. Bring patient to 'reality'. Talk quietly and slowly. Dialysis – strict asepsis when changing dialysate, catheter care. Check dialysate dwell time. Report slow return of fluid.
Dry mouth	Correct dehydration	Promote fluid intake to total of 3 litres per 24 hours. Oral hygiene two hourly.
Anorexia	Promote calorie intake to at least 2000 cal per 24 hr	Low-protein diet. High-carbohydrate diet (ascertain patient's preference). Serve food attractively. Add vitamins.
Nausea and vomiting Diarrhoea	See this unit	
Itching skin	Reduce blood urea Prevent skin infection	Keep fingernails short and clean. Bathe skin especially before sleeping. Use calamine lotion. Keep patient cool. Cotton clothes.
Tiredness and lethargy	Promote rest and sleep Increase oxygen carrying capacity of blood	Co-ordinate care to prevent tiring the patient. Ensure uninterrupted periods for rest and sleep. Care of blood transfusion. Monitor for any complications
	Prevent complications of bed rest by promoting mobility according to patient's ability.	Plantar flexion/extension. TED stockings. Wash legs. Deep breathing exercises. Inspect skin. Report breaks/redness. Prevent constipation. Aids to promote comfort. Promote personal hygiene.

Diet and **peritoneal dialysis** – even at home – may now extend these patients' lives considerably with continuous ambulatory peritoneal dialysis (CAPD). With the shortage of kidneys for transplantation, or if the patient cannot fulfil the requirement for a place in a haemodialysis programme, CAPD may sustain life until a donor kidney can be found, or improve their quality of life for the maximum time.

Activity

Examine diets reduced in protein available in your health district and explain how you would use them when preparing patients for discharge home.

3.7 Care of the patient with burns

Activity

Revise the structure and function of the skin (see Fig. 10.1, Unit 10). Burns and scalds are always the result of a tragic accident or an unbalanced mind, and the consequences can be horrific, causing terrible physical, emotional and social distress which may alter the person's whole life style.

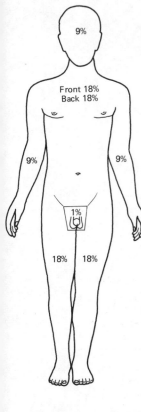

Burns are life threatening because of fluid imbalance. Fluid loss is proportional to the area of skin loss – the rule of nines (see Fig. 3.11). It is the loss of fluid, plasma protein and electrolytes that threaten life initially, causing profound shock. Later infection can cause septicaemia if strict attention is not paid to asepsis when dealing with the burned areas.

Pain is very severe in first-degree burns, but if the full thickness of the dermis is lost then nerve endings are lost. Pain is less severe, but although skin may be replaced by grafting, the sensation is lost in these grafted areas and this can be a potential hazard after recovery because the patient may be unaware of damage to the skin, e.g. sunburn, the area being against an extremely hot or cold object.

Assessment of the burned patient

1 Ascertain the level of consciousness. Is the airway clear?
2 When the burn occurred.
3 Nature of the agent causing the burn.
4 Length of exposure to burning agent (helps to establish depth of burn).
5 Any medications given prior to admission to hospital.
6 Whether heat or smoke has been inhaled.
7 Any pre-existing disease.
8 Normal weight prior to burn – helps in calculation of fluid loss and drug dosage.
9 Level of pain – severe pain can reduce blood pressure so increasing the depth of shock and the risk of acute renal failure. (Has analgesia been given at time of accident.)
10 Any known drug allergies.
11 Any likely associated injuries – head injuries, fractures.

Remember safe custody of valuables during emergency

Fig. 3.11
The rule of nines

Any clothing not adherent to body should be removed. Jewellery is removed especially from the hands before oedema becomes severe.

Assess the fluid imbalance

1 Moisture of tongue – degree of thirst (cells dehydrated).
2 Increasing restlessness = anxiety.
3 Rise in pulse rate = decreased blood volume.
4 Respiratory rate increased, rhythm normal – usually due to anxiety.
5 Blood pressure – profound shock.
     Do not sit patient up if shocked.
6 Cool pale skin – **unburned** area = compensatory vasoconstriction to maintain blood pressure.
7 Oliguria = decreased blood flow to the kidneys, increased ADH and aldosterone.
8 Convulsions may occur due to cerebral ischaemia.

Intravenous fluids administered to the burned patient may be:

1 Ringer's lactated solution – corrects acidosis, adds sodium.
2 Sodium bicarbonate 4.2%.
3 Isotonic saline – replaces lost sodium and water.
4 Plasma, dextran, plasma substitutes – raise blood volume, reduce shock.

The nurse **must** be alert to the dangers of giving **too much fluid too rapidly**, especially by IV infusion. These are:

1 Elevated CVP.
2 Shortness of breath – increased respiration, cough.
3 Increased blood pressure and pulse.
4 Anxiety.

Too little fluid or inadequate fluid replacement causes:

1 Decreased urinary output.
2 Elevated urinary specific gravity.
3 Decreased CVP.
4 Thirst.
5 Restlessness – disorientation.
6 Hypotension, increased pulse rate.

Danger! A patient with severe burns may develop:

1 Paralytic ileus nausea/vomiting/absence of bowel sounds.
2 Gastric dilatation.

Provide oral fluids only on the advice of medical staff. Because of thirst the patient is in danger of diluting body fluids if too much water is taken orally. **Water intoxication** is assessed by monitoring:

1 Headache
2 Depression
3 Apprehension
4 Tremors
5 Muscle twitching
6 Blurred vision
7 Vomiting
8 Diarrhoea
9 Disorientation
10 Excessive salivation
11 Mania
12 Generalized convulsion

Plain water or ice should be taken in limited amounts. Normal saline may be prescribed ORALLY disguised with flavouring or frozen as iced 'lolly'.

Average water loss from a major burn can amount to 2.5–4.0 litres per 24 hours.

Monitor urine output carefully

This may require catheterization. Assess hourly urine totals. Desired outputs per hour are 30–50 ml for men and 25–45 ml for women. For the causes and effects of acute renal failure, see Fig. 3.12.

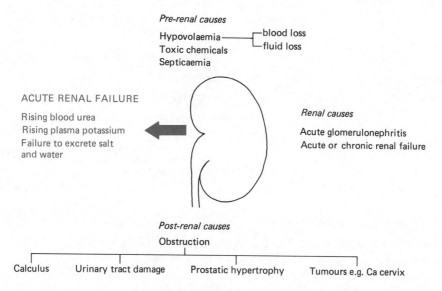

Fig. 3.12 Acute renal failure

Observe urine for clarity: damaged red cells in the body may result in haemoglobinuria; destroyed muscle may produce myoglobin.

Assess specific gravity.

Initial wound care

Analgesia/general anaesthesia required.

1 Do not prick blisters–they form effective sterile dressings.
2 Loose skin, dirt, etc are removed aseptically, often under anaesthesia.
3 Take swabs from sites of burns.
4 Cover with an occlusive non-adherent dressing.
5 Ensure antibiotic and tetanus cover.
6 Patient may be placed in reversed barrier isolation or in a side ward, to limit risk of infection.

Recovery phase

The patient will require increased dietary requirements: carbohydrates, protein; iron; vitamins.

For further details see Unit 2 if parenteral nutrition is required. See Unit 10 for a care plan for the patient with burns, and a discussion of the long-term patient problems.

3.8   Care of the patient with diarrhoea

Diarrhoea is a very distressing symptom, which, if severe, can be life threatening. The patient often complains of cramping abdominal pain, extreme lethargy and often the anal sphincter becomes sore and excoriated. The patient may be sweaty but feel cold and shiver.

The temperature may be elevated or below normal, depending upon the cause of the diarrhoea. The care of a patient with diarrhoea is discussed in Unit 6.

3.9   Care of the patient with fluid retention

Fig. 3.13 illustrates the causes and symptoms of overhydration.

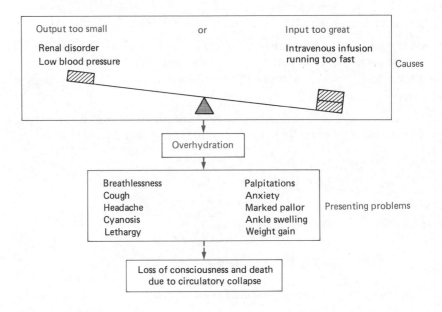

Fig. 3.13 Overhydration

The special needs of the patient receiving intravenous fluids

1 The patient must know why the fluids are required; the nurse should explain.
2 Promotion of comfort is important during the infusion.
   (a) Ensure clothing is easily changed.
   (b) Support the limb – avoid dominant arm if possible.
   (c) Ensure siting of infusion will facilitate maximum movement. A frozen shoulder can result from immobility if exercise of shoulder muscles is not encouraged.
3 Observe for evidence of inflammation at cannula site:
   change giving sets daily;
   ensure sterility when changing infusion bags (see Fig. 3.14 opposite);
   an occlusive dressing at the cannula site is preferred.
4 Ensure the correct fluid is given – check as stated in local district policy. Fluid should be checked at the bedside with the treatment card, also for expiry date, clarity of fluid, batch number and that the container is not damaged in any way.
5 Remember to chart fluid commenced on fluid chart (see fluid chart in Appendix)

In situations of severe fluid imbalance the monitoring of central venous pressure is undertaken, and the nurse is responsible for taking and recording the readings.

Activity

What three factors aid blood to return to the heart via the venous system?

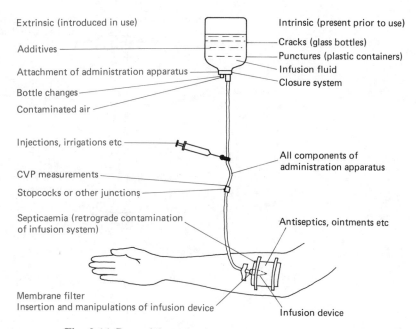

Extrinsic (introduced in use)
Additives
Attachment of administration apparatus
Bottle changes
Contaminated air
Injections, irrigations etc
CVP measurements
Stopcocks or other junctions
Septicaemia (retrograde contamination of infusion system)
Membrane filter
Insertion and manipulations of infusion device

Intrinsic (present prior to use)
Cracks (glass bottles)
Punctures (plastic containers)
Infusion fluid
Closure system
All components of administration apparatus
Antiseptics, ointments etc
Infusion device

Fig. 3.14 Potential mechanisms for contamination during intravenous infusion

Central venous pressure

What is central venous pressure? It is the pressure of blood in the large veins and the right atrium of the heart. Normally this pressure is low $(0-10$ cm $H_2O)$ because the blood is returning to the heart and the resistance of the blood vessels has slowed down the blood flow.

A cannula is placed so that the tip is in the right atrium of the heart (see Fig. 3.15). This enables blood pressure readings to be measured within the circulation. A special intravenous giving set which has a manometer attached to it, enables this pressure of blood to support a column of water (centimetres of water pressure). Normal pressure $= 0-10$ cm H_2O (see Fig. 3.16 overleaf).

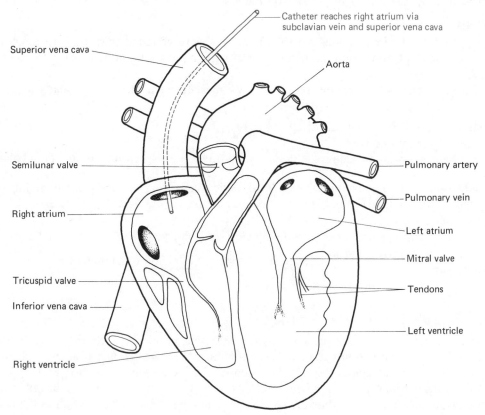

Catheter reaches right atrium via subclavian vein and superior vena cava
Superior vena cava
Aorta
Semilunar valve
Right atrium
Tricuspid valve
Inferior vena cava
Right ventricle
Pulmonary artery
Pulmonary vein
Left atrium
Mitral valve
Tendons
Left ventricle

Fig. 3.15 Position of catheter during central venous pressure measurement

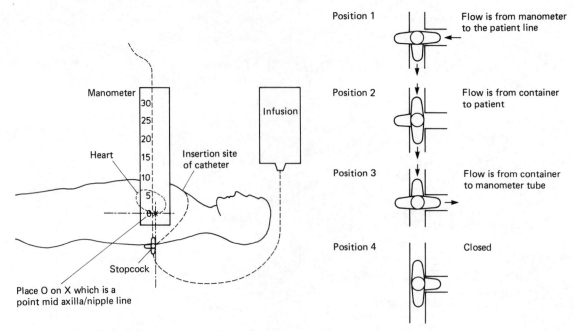

Fig. 3.16 Measurement of central venous pressure

It is important when making the readings that the scale for measuring the CVP is checked each time, and that 0 is at the same level as the right atrium.

Activity

Why is this level important? What would be the result of the reading if:

1 The scale was higher than the right atrium?
2 The right atrium was lower than 0 on the scale?
3 The scale was lower than the right atrium?
4 The right atrium was higher than 0 on the scale?

Activity

What would be the implications for treatment if it were assumed that these readings were accurate? How can you ensure accuracy? Identify the equipment and learn how to check the levels.

If you are caring for a patient requiring CVP measurement then ensure that you know:

1 The reason for measuring CVP.
2 How to record the CVP accurately.
3 What to report and why.
4 The significance of recording the pulse, blood pressure, respiration, colour, fluid balance.

Consult your own nursing notes and local policy regarding changing CVP giving sets, especially if the cannula is sited via the subclavian vein.

Dangers of cannulation

Air embolus – this is a danger each time a giving set is changed.
Erosion of great blood vessels ⎫ especially during introduction of cannula.
Pneumothorax ⎭
Septicaemia – strict asepsis necessary.

3.10   Care of the patient with advanced liver failure

The patient with liver failure presents many distressing problems, including disturbance of fluid balance. Not all patients have all the problems, therefore a careful assessment of the patient's physical and emotional state is essential. The patient's social background is also important because advanced liver failure usually indicates an inability to work or take care of the family, and patients of a relatively young age group may be affected, as well as the middle and older age groups.

Activity

Revise the functions of the liver.

Care plan for a patient with liver failure

Problem	Aim	Nursing care
Weakness, fatigue	Promote rest Prevent pressure sores	Rest and activity as desired. Provide suitable aids to promote comfort. Turn patient two hourly. Norton scale.
Anorexia, nausea, vomiting, diarrhoea or constipation	Promote appetite and minimize weight loss Prevent any infections	Keep mouth fresh and clean with soft brush. High-carbohydrate diet. Low- protein diet. Low-salt diet. Monitor stools for blood. Particular attention to personal hygiene due to reduced immunity. Monitor temperature and pulse rate.
Abdominal fullness, flatulence, ascites, enlarged liver and spleen	Ease discomfort of abdominal distension and aid respirations	Keep well supported in bed – upright position. Chair may provide alternative place to rest. Paracentesis abdominus may be performed. Drain fluid very slowly. Monitor respirations.
Oedema	Prevent circulatory overload	May restrict fluid intake. Distribute intake during waking hours to reduce discomfort. Monitor all fluid intake/output. Monitor blood pressure.
Jaundice – skin may itch due to bile pigments in skin, also urine dark due to bile	Alleviate itching	Avoid patient having a mirror if jaundice very severe. Bath at night to promote rest/sleep. Gloves may prevent scratching. Keep finger nails clean. Be sensitive to needs of patient and visitors.
Bruising, bleeding gums, severe bleeding from gastro-intestinal tract	Assess for haemorrhage	Avoid injections. Inspect faeces for blood. Inspect vomit for blood. Remove any blood from bowel with enema if necessary.
Dullness, loss of memory, slow speech, personality changes, confusion, may lead to coma	Monitor behavioural changes	Monitor level of consciousness, moodswings, hand flapping, ability to concentrate.
	Promote self-esteem of patient	Provide information and encourage patient decisions. Listen to worries and fears. Provide support from other professionals. Encourage family to assist with care.

Other patient problems apart from those in the care plan include:

1 Low-grade pyrexia (feeling hot or cold).
2 Faecal odour to breath.
3 Spider angiomata – dilated superficial blood vessels.
4 Enlarged breasts in the male patient and atrophy of the testicles owing to an inability to deactivate oestrogen.
5 Hyperventilation if blood ammonia levels are high – due to liver's inability to convert ammonia to urea for excretion by the kidney. Ammonia levels are especially elevated if bleeding in the gastro-intestinal tract occurs. The blood proteins in the gastro-intestinal tract are digested and absorbed, in turn causing ammonia levels to rise.
6 Deficiency in vitamins A and B may cause problems with vision and the skin as the liver cannot store them. A sore mouth, bleeding gums and a reduced ability to heal result.
7 Adverse effects from medications may occur as the liver cannot detoxify drugs and therefore they cannot be excreted.
8 Recurrent infection due to decreased formation of antibodies. **Prevention** of infection is very important.

In this unit we are considering fluid imbalance. For care of the patient who is haemorrhaging and breathless, please refer to Units 4 and 5.

Activity

Refer to the diagram demonstrating how the body fluids are distributed in normal health (Fig. 3.5) and modify it to demonstrate a lowered osmotic pressure of plasma proteins and a raised blood pressure in the venules. You should now be able to explain why the patient with liver failure becomes oedematous, and may develop ascites. Consult your tutor if you find this difficult.

Activity

Revise the portal circulation by asking yourself:

1 Where does the liver receive its blood supply from?

2 What are the implications for food digested in the gastro-intestinal tract in patients with portal congestion, in relation to:
Absorption in the villi of the small intestine?
Propulsion of food through the bowel?

3 What signs and symptoms may the patient demonstrate, if he has severe internal bleeding?
4 What action would you take?

The patient and family will require much emotional support, and the nursing team need to be available to:

1 Provide information about the patient's condition.
2 Be prepared to listen to their fears and anxieties.
3 Contact a social worker if the family requires social support.
4 Contact the general practitioner if the family's health becomes a cause for concern.
5 Children, particularly adolescents in the family, may be especially disturbed when a parent is ill.

Activity

Who can assist adolescents during the illness of a parent? How may the children react to the illness?

3.11 Care of the patient with nephrotic syndrome

Nephrotic syndrome is a kidney condition in which the glomerulus of the kidney allows protein – especially albumin – through the glomerular capsule into the filtrate. Because of this abnormal loss of protein in the urine, the plasma protein levels fall, so reducing the osmotic pressure of the blood. Fluid passes to the tissues of the body, but it then is unable to return back to the circulation. Marked generalized oedema results, and 30 – 40 g protein may be lost daily.

Activity

Return to the diagram on formation of tissue fluid (page 22). Alter the diagram to demonstrate how oedema is formed when plasma proteins are reduced. Consult your tutor if you have a problem (see Fig. 3.17).

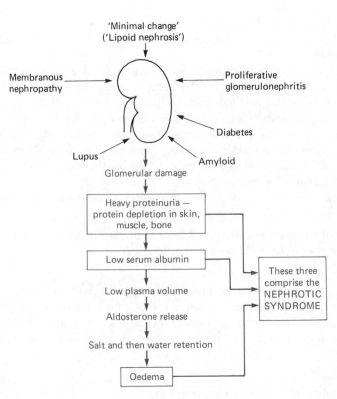

Fig. 3.17 Nephrotic syndrome

Causes of nephrotic syndrome

These include:

1 Inflammatory renal disease (acute glomerular nephritis).
2 Glomerular disease associated with systemic diseases – systemic lupus erythematosis, amyloidosis and diabetes.
3 Mechanical disorders:
   thrombosis of the renal vein
   poisons affecting the kidney, e.g. mercury
   renal transplantation

Assessment of the patient with nephrotic syndrome

1 How long has the patient felt unwell? Ask about previous illnesses.
2 Is there a history of sore throats?
3 For how long has the patient noticed swelling of the body?
4 Visual assessment:
   Is the oedema generalized; dependent; pitting?
   In male patients is the penis oedematous? (This may cause difficulty in passing urine.)
   Are the eyelids oedematous?
   Measure the girth – is there ascites?
   Respiratory rate – is breathlessness a problem?
   Assess the state of the patient's tongue and mouth.
   Is the patient thirsty?
5 Weigh the patient accurately.
6 Assess the patient's cerebral function – headache, level of consciousness.

Symptoms of cerebral oedema are bradycardia, hypertension, pyrexia and slow, deep respirations. The age of the patient requires consideration when looking at normal levels.

REPORT ANY ABNORMALITIES IMMEDIATELY

This renal condition may resolve spontaneously or may proceed to chronic renal failure. Children with this condition are more likely to recover than adults. The severity of symptoms is very variable, and therefore the following care plan will need to be modified according to the individual needs of the patient. Adrenal corticosteroids may be used to decrease proteinuria and increase urinary output, though it is not clear how they work.

Care plan for a patient with nephrotic syndrome

Patient problem	Aim	Nursing care
Headache	Assess cause of headache	Assess location and intensity of headache, mental state and level of consciousness. Reduce light and noise levels.
Extreme lethargy	Promote rest and comfort	Select aids to promote comfort. Turn patient two hourly. Inspect pressure areas for redness and breaks in skin.
Breathlessness and marked oedema	Reduce oedema Maintain personal hygiene	Position upright. Ensure skin not pulled when changing position, etc. Skin may tear easily if oedema severe (care needed if blood pressure recorded). Mouth care. Ensure patient's skin dry in skin folds. Swollen eyelids – bathe eyes two hourly. May be oedematous.
Anorexia	Promote high protein intake	Dietician/medical staff calculate protein intake. IV albumin may be administered. Care of infusion and watch for adverse reaction.
Reduced immunity	Prevent infection	Screen staff for colds, etc. Nurse in side ward if possible. Protective isolation may be necessary. Monitor body temperature, pulse.

For a quick and easy revision test on this unit turn to page 110.

Further reading

Baker, J. and Boore, J., 'Fluids in balance' (*Nursing*, 1st series, no 13, all articles, May 1980)
Cameron, J. S. and Russell, A. M., *Nephrology for Nurses* (Heinemann Medical Books Ltd, 1970)
Cooke, S. M., 'Heart Failure' (*Nursing*, 1st series, no 33, January 1982), 1435

Donovan, M. and Schrober J., 'Hypertension' (*Nursing*, 1st series, January 1982), 1431

Ginsburg, J. and Fink, R. S., 'Diabetes Mellitus' (*Nursing*, vol 2, no 13, May 1983), 369

Goodinson, S. M., 'Shock' (*Nursing*, 1st series, no 33, January 1982), 1440

Goodinson, S. M., 'Coronary Artery Disease' (*Nursing*, 2nd series, no 25, May 1984) 732

Green, S. P., 'Deep Vein Thrombosis' (*Nursing*, 1st series, no 33, January 1982), 1468

Hancock, H. M., 'Circulation – an overview' (*Nursing*, vol 2, no 25, May 1984), 726

Hayward, J., 'Information – a Prescription for Pain' (RCN, 1975)

Herbert, R., 'Maintaining the Circulatory Volume' (*Nursing*, vol 2, no 26, June 1984), 766

Heslip, M. C., 'Burns Injuries' (*Nursing*, vol 2, no 11, March 1983)

Kitchen, I., 'Congestive Heart Failure' (*Nursing*, vol 2, no 25, May 1984)

'Personal View', 'Myocardial Infarction' (*Nursing*, vol 2, no 25, May 1984), 737

'Personal View', 'Myocardial Infarction (Rehabilitation)' (*Nursing*, vol 2, no 25, May 1984), 740

4 Care of the breathless patient

4.1 Important points when nursing the breathless patient

Reassurance

The greatest problems faced by the breathless patient are **fear and anxiety**. Whatever the cause of breathlessness this is a common problem and is therefore dealt with as a subject in its own right. Nurses commonly deal with this 'problem' in their answers by writing 'reassure the patient'. What we need to know is *How*? The presence of another person who is calm and appears to be in control is very helpful. See Section I for more details concerning this problem.

Practical details

Nursing measures to minimize the problems of breathlessness and promote effective ventilation of the lungs are important, not only to minimize the problem, but also to enable the nurse to gain the patient's confidence.

 1 Place the patient in the most comfortable position – usually upright.
 2 Facilitate chest expansion – prevent shoulders leaning forward.
 3 Administer oxygen **as prescribed on the prescription sheet**.
 4 Minimize anxiety and movement of the patient to reduce oxygen demand. Keep your voice calm and explain procedures carefully to the patient.
 5 Discourage the patient from speaking. – Ask 'closed questions' to prevent distress when talking. (See Appendix, page 147).
 6 Promote ventilation of the bed area.   7 Provide light cotton bedclothes.
 8 Keep the mouth fresh and clean, providing oral hygiene according to the patient's needs.

Before considering in detail the specific care of the breathless patient, study of the causes of breathlessness is essential to understanding nursing care and medical treatment.

4.2 The respiratory system

Activity

Study the structure of the respiratory system and identify the functions of the upper respiratory tract. What is meant by the term 'dead space'? Where does respiration take place in the body? How does respiration occur? (See Figs 4.1 and 4.2.)

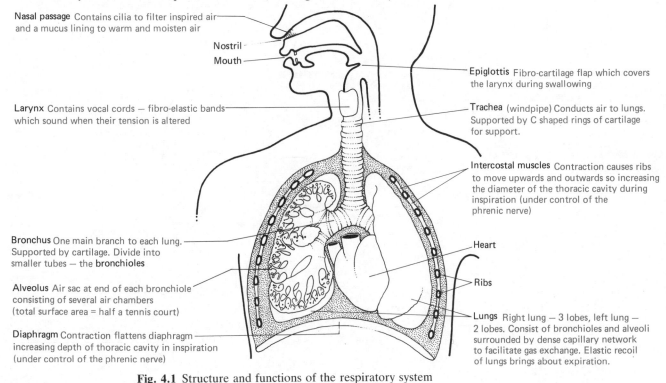

Nasal passage Contains cilia to filter inspired air and a mucus lining to warm and moisten air

Nostril

Mouth

Epiglottis Fibro-cartilage flap which covers the larynx during swallowing

Larynx Contains vocal cords — fibro-elastic bands which sound when their tension is altered

Trachea (windpipe) Conducts air to lungs. Supported by C shaped rings of cartilage for support.

Intercostal muscles Contraction causes ribs to move upwards and outwards so increasing the diameter of the thoracic cavity during inspiration (under control of the phrenic nerve)

Bronchus One main branch to each lung. Supported by cartilage. Divide into smaller tubes — the bronchioles

Heart

Ribs

Alveolus Air sac at end of each bronchiole consisting of several air chambers (total surface area = half a tennis court)

Lungs Right lung — 3 lobes, left lung — 2 lobes. Consist of bronchioles and alveoli surrounded by dense capillary network to facilitate gas exchange. Elastic recoil of lungs brings about expiration.

Diaphragm Contraction flattens diaphragm increasing depth of thoracic cavity in inspiration (under control of the phrenic nerve)

Fig. 4.1 Structure and functions of the respiratory system

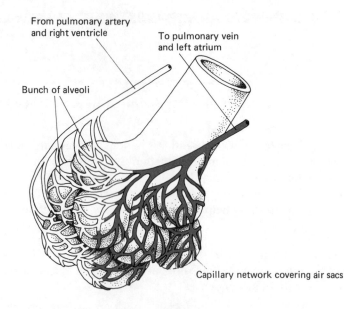

Fig. 4.2 Structure of the alveoli

The mechanism of respiration

During respiration the size of the thoracic cavity increases. This is brought about by the contraction of the diaphragm and the intercostal muscles (see Fig. 4.3).

In the upright position the abdominal contents fall away from the diaphragm, so facilitating inspiration.

In quiet breathing approximately 500 ml of atmospheric air are inspired in a single breath, but only 250 ml of this air actually reach the alveoli due to the filling of the nasal passages, the pharynx, the trachea and the bronchi (the 'dead space' where gas exchange cannot take place). Table 4.1 shows how the composition of air changes during respiration.

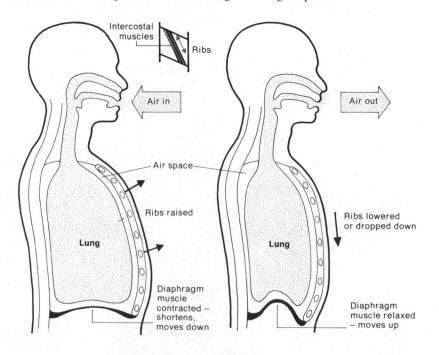

Fig. 4.3 Mechanism of respiration

Table 4.1 Percentages of gases in inspired and expired air

Atmospheric air	Inspired air	Expired air
Oxygen	20.95%	16.4%
Nitrogen	79.00%	79.5%
Carbon dioxide	00.4%	4.0%

Respiratory gases are exchanged in the alveoli – **external respiration** (see Fig. 4.4). Gases in solution are exchanged in the tissues – **internal respiration** (see Fig. 4.5). The process of gaseous exchange is by **diffusion**, i.e. movement of gas from a high concentration to a lower concentration.

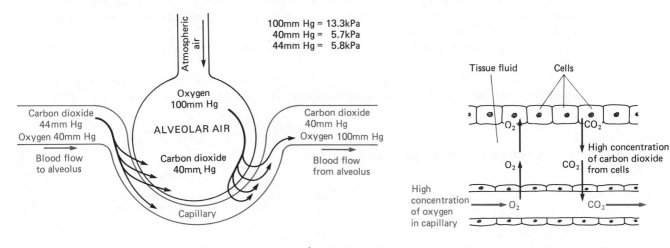

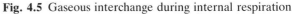

Fig. 4.4 Gaseous interchange in the alveolus – external respiration

Fig. 4.5 Gaseous interchange during internal respiration

The nervous control of respiration (see Figs. 4.6 and 4.7)

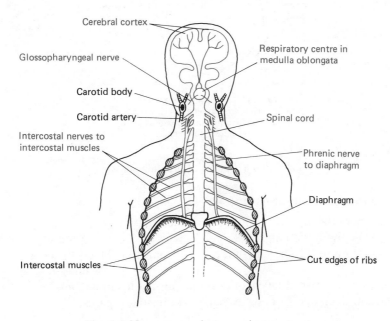

Fig. 4.6 Nervous supply to respiratory tract

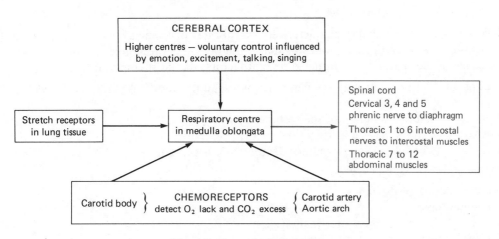

Fig. 4.7 Control of respiration

The respiratory centre in the medulla oblongata is normally stimulated by raised levels of carbon dioxide in the blood. If persons suffer from a chronic respiratory disease they have a permanently raised level of carbon dioxide and the respiratory centre is no longer stimulated by carbon dioxide but by lack of oxygen. To administer a high concentration of oxygen would reduce the respiration rate and depth, and carbon dioxide levels rise in the blood (RESPIRATORY ACIDOSIS). This lowering of the blood pH eventually inhibits the nervous system, heart and lungs from functioning. Death results.

Compression of the respiratory centre, e.g. head injury, will also slow and deepen respiration.

Transection of the spinal cord at level $C_1 - C_2$ will inactivate the nerve supply to the diaphragm and intercostal muscles. Respiratory arrest will occur. Artificial ventilation will be required.

4.3   Causes of breathlessness (see Fig. 4.8)

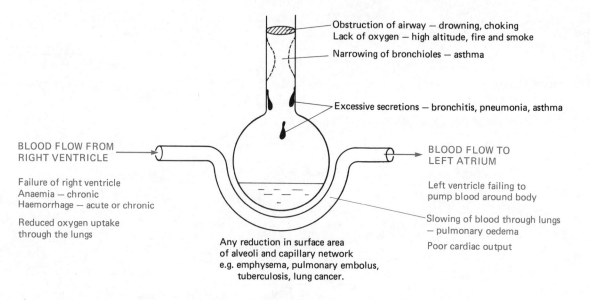

Fig. 4.8 Causes of breathlessness

For normal respiration you must have:

1 Good air entry to the alveoli – ventilation of the lungs.
2 Good blood supply to the lungs.
   Good blood return to the left side of the heart from the lungs. } Perfusion of blood through the lungs.
3 Blood able to carry normal levels of oxygen – normal haemoglobin.
4 Healthy alveoli to enable gaseous exchange – diffusion of gases.

4.4   Care of the patient with asthma

Asthma is a condition that is characterized by episodes of bronchospasm and spasm of the bronchioles. Between these episodes of spasm the person is often able to breathe normally. The cause of the spasm may be due to several factors, the most common being:

1 Exposure to foreign protein – pollen, dust, house mites, foods. ASSESS ALL PATIENTS FOR ALLERGENS.
2 Viral or bacterial infection of the respiratory tract.
3 Anxiety or stress may be a triggering factor.
4 Cause may be unknown. Hereditary factor often is present.

Complications of asthma are:

1 Overinflation of the lungs.
2 Pneumothorax.
3 Widespread emphysema after many years.
4 Infection with Aspergillus – a fungus.

Method of grading the severity of asthma

Grade IA
Some difficulty in carrying out job or housework.
Sleep occasionally disturbed.
Asthma relieved by inhaler.

Grade IB
Job or housework carried out with great difficulty.
Sleep frequently disturbed.
Inhaler of limited use.

Grade IIA
Patient confined to chair or bed, but can get up for short periods, e.g. to make a cup of tea.
Sleep very disturbed.
Inhaler of no use at all.

Grade IIB
Patient confined to chair or bed and can get up only with great difficulty.
Sleep impossible.
Pulse rate 120 per minute or more.

Grade III
Patient totally confined to bed or chair.
Pulse rate 120 per minute or more.

Grade IV
Complete exhaustion.
Pulse rate 120 per minute or more.

Preparation of the bed area for a patient with asthma

1 Remove all flowers from the environment.
2 Make sure pillows are foam not feather.
3 Oxygen – give high concentration unless otherwise prescribed.
4 A fan may assist circulation of air in the bed area – ensure flex and fan blades are safe.
5 Equipment to monitor blood pressure and TPR will be needed.
6 Obtain previous notes and X-rays if available.

Assessment of the patient's physical state

1 Monitor respiratory rate.
2 Monitor pulse rate – if 120 beats per min or over (adult) there is danger of heart failure.
3 Patient's colour – dark brown/pale brown/grey-brown in negroes. Pink, pallor, grey, cyanosed.
4 Patient's skin – warm/cold; warm/wet; cold and sweating.
5 Is the patient exhausted? Confused?
6 How long has the patient been distressed?
7 What medication has been given?
8 Monitor the blood pressure – if it is lowered this may indicate heart failure.
9 Monitor temperature in axilla.

Obtain social details from a relative if possible.
   The nurse's responsibilities are to monitor the effect of medication and report any changes that occur.
   Drugs that may be given are:

1 Aminophylline, intravenous route – danger of hypotension.
2 Adrenaline – danger of tachycardia.
3 Steroids – intravenously, or as an inhalation, via a nebulizer.
4 Antibiotics.
5 Monitor the intravenous infusion flow rate to ensure that the circulation is not overloaded.
6 Keep the patient comfortable and minimize exertion.

When bronchospasm has been relieved

1 Promote comfort – change sheets and nightwear as required. Ensure the skin is clean and dry.

2 Promote fluid intake – give high-calorie drinks.
3 Enable the patient to rest.
4 Co-ordinate care to prevent the patient becoming overtired.

For a patient's first attack of asthma a sociological assessment is needed:

1 Home – possible allergens, problems with relationships.
2 Occupation (including school).
3 Hobbies (sports, etc).

Prior to discharge the patient may be prescribed drugs to:

1 Prevent bronchospasm – Ventolin (salbutamol) or Intal (sodium cromoglycate).
2 Prevent respiratory infection – long-term antibiotics.
3 Reduce bronchospasm and oedema – Ventolin or steroids by inhaler.

The patient must know:

1 How to use the inhalers.
2 What the different inhalants are prescribed for.
3 When to take the drugs and their possible side-effects.
4 They must carry a steroid card.

4.5 Care of the patient with excessive sputum

Examples are the patient with chronic bronchitis or pneumonia.

Care plan for the patient with excessive sputum

Problem	Aim of care	Nursing care
Inability to breathe especially on exertion	Remove sputum	Position upright.
	Increase pulmonary ventilation and oxygenation of blood	Moist inhalations followed by chest physiotherapy – drainage, percussion. Provide sputum pot and tissues. Send specimen of sputum to laboratory. Take peak flow readings. Administer oxygen as prescribed. Monitor respiratory rate; ensure use of accessory muscles.
	Monitor for evidence of heart failure. Reduce infection	Look for evidence of oedema in sacrum and ankles. Monitor blood pressure – hypertension. Monitor for side-effects of antibiotics.
Dry mouth due to inability to eat and drink	Correct dehydration Keep mouth moist	Small frequent drinks. IV infusion may be necessary – watch for danger of circulatory overload. Oral hygiene as necessary.
Anorexia	Prevent constipation	Ensure bowel action – ascertain whether any constipation present.
Reduced mobility	Prevent complications of bed rest	Turn two hourly. Use aids to spread pressure. Monitor pressure areas for redness. Use Norton scale (see Appendix). Check legs for tenderness and oedema.
Pyrexia	Maintain normal body temperature	Tepid sponge patient. Fan – avoid chilling. Cotton nightwear. Four hourly TPR.
Tiredness and fatigue	Promote rest and sleep	Coordinate care ensuring rest. DO NOT SEDATE PATIENTS WITH CHRONIC BRONCHITIS.
Confusion	Ensure patient safety	No smoking signs. Low bed – avoid cot sides if possible. Reorientate patient gradually. Ensure continuity of staff to patient if possible. Keep voice calm. Avoid darkened environment.

Antibiotics do not remove sputum from the alveoli, so it is vital that effective chest physiotherapy removes the sputum and increases pulmonary ventilation.

Assisting the patient to remove sputum

1 Provide moist inhalation – do not leave a patient unattended with **steam** inhalation.
2 Change position two hourly enabling the patient to lie as low as tolerable prior to physiotherapy and coughing.
3 Encourage EXHALATION as far as possible. This often triggers the cough reflex.
4 Avoid physiotherapy after meals – the patient may vomit the meal – immediately before meals and just before visiting – as these may cause exhaustion.

Advice to patients on discharge

1 Avoid irritants to respiratory tract – smoking, pollutants from industry, the home, garden and farming.
2 Avoid extreme cold – the bedroom should be warm but ventilated (a heating allowance may be available).
3 Exercise within the limits of the individual.
4 Prevent obesity.
5 Report any increase in breathlessness and ankle swelling to the general practitioner.
6 Take medication (long-term antibiotics during the winter) as prescribed by the doctor.
7 Avoid crowds and people with respiratory infections.
8 Influenza vaccination may be offered.

Breathlessness may occur in diseases of the lung, where tissue has been destroyed, and the surface area for gaseous exchange is reduced. These diseases are:

1 **Emphysema** – often a complication of chronic bronchitis and asthma.
2 **Lung cancer** – often discovered as 'pneumonia'.
3 **Tuberculosis** – an inflammatory infectious state and weight loss.
4 **Cystic fibrosis** – excessive tenacious secretions of the lungs.

The problems the patient may experience are often very similar to those of patients with excessive secretions:

1 Pyrexia – see Unit 7.
2 Infection – may require isolation procedure.

Activity

1 Read the care of patients with the above diseases.
2 Identify the patient's actual and potential problems and construct a care plan for: the acute stage of the illness; advice prior to discharge home; a patient following pneumonectomy for lung cancer.
3 Look up the preparation and care for a patient receiving a course of radiotherapy and of cytotoxic therapy.

4 Identify organizations who provide assistance to families with children with cystic fibrosis. How are these patients cared for in the community? What are the implications for the family? What increased responsibilities do they have with the care of the patient? How is the disease transmitted?

4.6   Care of the anaemic patient

Fig. 4.9 revises the production (erythropoiesis), circulation and destruction of red blood cells. Breathlessness may be due to:

1 A reduced number of red blood cells due to decreased production in the bone marrow; acute or chronic blood loss.
2 A reduced amount of haemoglobin in red cells.
3 Misshapen red cells – sickle cell anaemia.
4 Increased destruction of red cells.

Fig. 4.10 shows the different types of anaemias. In all cases the blood has a reduced ability to carry normal levels of oxygen.

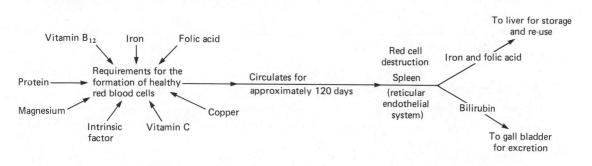

Fig. 4.9 Production (erythropoiesis), circulation and destruction of red blood cells

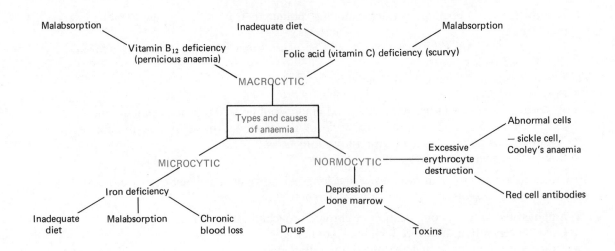

Fig. 4.10 Types and causes of anaemia

Care plan for the patient with anaemia

Problem	Aim of care	Nursing care
Breathlessness on exertion	Reduce oxygen requirements of the body	Bed rest in position most comfortable for the patient. Administer oxygen as prescribed if required. Oral hygiene to prevent dry mouth. No smoking signs to ensure patient's safety.
Tiredness and lethargy	Prevent complication of bed rest	Change position two hourly. Provide aids to comfort and prevent pressure sores (see Appendix). Assess Norton scale. Observe legs for tenderness in the calves and ankle oedema. Give high-fibre diet to prevent constipation.
Poor appetite	Provide diet containing essential ingredients for red blood cell production	Diet should be high in iron, vitamin C, protein, vitamin B_{12}, folic acid and trace elements. Arrange small meals in an appetizing form – assess food preferences. Assess nutritional state. Supplement meals as required.

Specific care for differing causes of anaemia

1 Iron deficiency anaemia:
   (a) Chronic blood loss. Observe stools, urine, menstrual loss, bruising, haemorrhoids, epistaxis.
   (b) Acute blood loss. Blood transfusion – see Unit 5. Treat with iron therapy.
2 Scurvy (lack of vitamin C): assess dietary intake and cooking methods. Observe for bruising and tenderness of long bones and joints. Ability to heal is reduced – protect extremities, etc.
3 Pernicious anaemia: monitor neurological state – numbness, tingling of extremities. Injection of vitamin B_{12} for life will be necessary.
4 Increased destruction of red cells: jaundice (see Unit 3.10).
5 Inability to absorb nutrients from the intestine: carry out nutritional assessment; may be an X-ray examination of the intestinal tract; assess weight regularly (nutritional supplements may be required) (see Unit 2.6).
6 Inability to produce red cells in sufficient quantities (leukaemia): reversal barrier isolation; blood transfusion; cytotoxic therapy.

4.7   Care of the patient with congestive heart failure

Before considering the care of the patient, an understanding of the causes of the disease is necessary in order to be able to assess the patient's needs and identify the actual and potential problems.

Congestive heart failure is often due to two main factors:

1 A chronic respiratory disorder – chronic bronchitis or emphysema.
2 A long-term failure of the left ventricle.

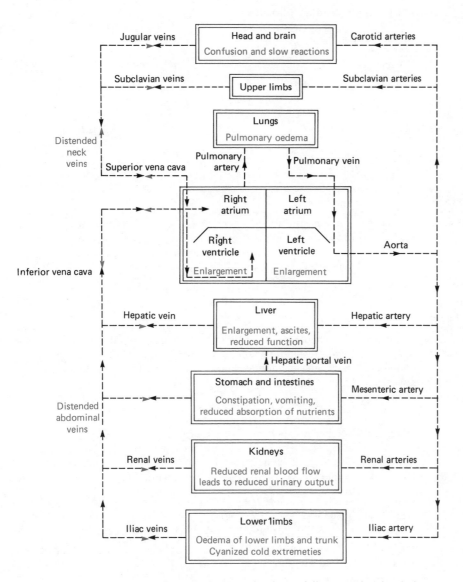

Fig. 4.11 Effects of congestive heart failure on the circulation

In both situations a rise in blood pressure occurs in the lungs causing the right ventricle to pump harder against the increased pressure in the lungs. Congestion of all venous blood ultimately occurs as the right ventricle fails. Fig. 4.11 shows the circulation and effects of congestive heart failure.

Diuretics gradually reduce the circulatory volume and breathlessness and gastro-intestinal problems decline. The fluid balance chart (see Appendix) must be maintained accurately and the patient weighed daily (see Unit 3). Mobility is gradually increased and the patient gradually resumes responsibility for the problems of daily living.

Prior to discharge the patient will need to understand:

1 Medication – Why it needs to be taken regularly.
   What to report to the doctor or nurse – breathlessness, increasing oedema.
   Increasing lethargy   ⎫ side-effects of
   Nausea and vomiting   ⎬ digoxin toxicity and
   Disturbances of vision   ⎭ potassium depletion

2 Need to exercise within personal limits.

3 Avoid cold.

The patient may need care and support from the following groups of people in the community and hospital, especially if they live alone:

General practitioner – medication
District nurse or bath assistant – monitor total patient needs

Health visitor ⎫
Social worker ⎬ pensions, supplementary allowances
⎭
Meals on wheels
Home help
Chiropodist
Day hospital
Ambulance service
Hospital consultant
Family and neighbours

Care plan for the patient with congestive heart failure

Problem	Aim of care	Nursing care
Difficulty in breathing in upright position	Increase oxygen levels to the brain and heart muscle	Nurse at complete rest. Upright position well supported with pillow. Monitor respiration, pulse and blood pressure hourly. Administer oxygen – low concentration; safety signs for patient safety. Oral toilet to prevent dry mouth. Keep face dry and cool.
Oedema (pitting of the legs)	Reduce circulatory volume by increasing urinary output	Monitor the effect of diuretic drugs – fluid balance chart (see Appendix). Restrict fluid intake. Reduce sodium intake.
Extreme anxiety and pain (angina, enlarged liver and ascites)	To reduce immediate stress and reduce heart rate To reduce intra-abdominal pressure and drain ascites if present	Morphine sulphate is often drug of choice – monitor respiratory rate for any respiratory depression. Monitor pulse and blood pressure. Paracentesis abdominus – monitor vital body systems for shock. Drain fluid slowly.
Reduced mobility	Prevent complications of bed rest	Assess on Norton scale (see Appendix). Aids to distribute body weight due to oedema: large cell ripple mattress; or air ring; sheepskin on heels and elbows; bed cradle. Bed that facilitates lowering the legs may assist breathing for the distressed patient. Monitor legs for evidence of deep-vein thrombosis. Turn, change position two hourly.
Nausea/vomiting	Keep mouth fresh and clean	Use anti-emetic drugs. Discreet placement of vomit bowl and tissues. Reduce sodium intake (including soda water).
Anorexia	Provide calorie intake to prevent muscle breakdown	Assess preferences of light meals (restrict fluid). Add carbohydrate as tolerated by patient.
Constipation	Prevent constipation, or relieve it if present	Ensure the bowel is clear of impacted faeces. Ensure regular bowel action. Haemorrhoids may be present and painful. Commode often most comfortable for the patient and facilitates too the emptying of the bladder.
Promotion of personal hygiene	To promote the well-being of the patient	To assist with personal hygiene according to patient's need, ensuring all skin surfaces are clean and dry. Hair may require washing or use dry shampoo as sweating makes hair unattractive.

4.8   Care of the patient with acute left ventricular failure

This is an acute medical emergency, and can lead to cardiac arrest if not controlled effectively by the nurse taking prompt action immediately and assisting with medical treatment.

Care plan for a patient with acute left ventricular failure

Problem	Aim of care	Nursing care
Acute distress due to difficulty with breathing Cough and frothy sputum Pallor/cyanosis	Increase of oxygenation of blood Improve ventilation Decrease circulatory volume	MEDICAL EMERGENCY. Call for medical help – stay with patient. Sit him up. Monitor blood pressure and pulse. Keep calm. Give high percentage oxygen. Prepare for administration of diurectics and possible sedation.

Care plan (*continued*)

Problem	Aim of care	Nursing care
Extreme fear	Reduce anxiety to reduce heart activity Identify cause of complication immediately	Monitor patient's colour and state of skin. Monitor level of consciousness. Observe pupil size/convulsive movements; carotid pulse present. Assist with ECG. Observe safety regulation – chest X-ray with portable machine. Monitor urinary output and respiratory rate in response to diuretic therapy.
Excessive sweating	Keep skin dry and promote rest	Remove nightwear sheets as necessary. Keep mouth moist. Remove from sight any equipment that may cause alarm. Stay within vision of the patient to provide feeling of security. Promote sleep.
Chest pain may be a problem	Reduce pain/provide analgesia	Monitor response to analgesia – IV venflon may be *in situ* to administer drugs.

The problem of breathlessness is due to stagnation of the blood in the lungs due to failure of the left ventricle of the heart to maintain the systemic blood flow (see Fig. 4.12).

This emergency situation is frightening for the patient, the nurse and relatives, because if the situation cannot be reversed death may result.

Relatives are often 'called in' by telephone and naturally they are very anxious and distressed. Bewilderment may be another reaction because the patient seemed to be making a marvellous recovery after a 'heart attack'. 'Why has it happened nurse?' and 'He will get better won't he?' are common questions from relatives. It is best to be truthful and the following advice has been useful to me personally.

First, nobody can predict a 'heart attack', but some factors are known to increase the risks. Once the patient has survived the initial heart damage then he or she requires rest until the heart has had time to heal. Ascertain if there are any known problems, for example worries regarding the family, work, etc which may be causing anxiety.

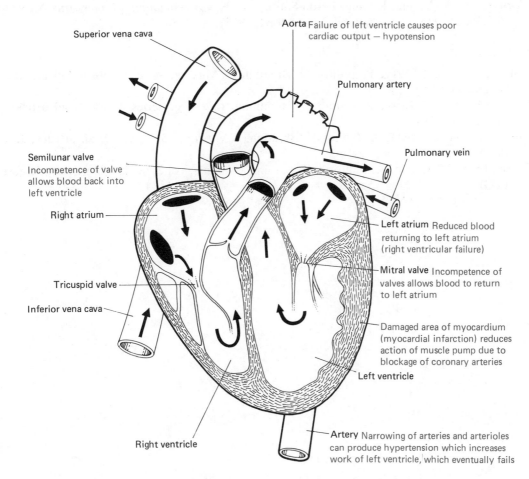

Fig. 4.12 Causes of left ventricular failure

Secondly, the question 'He will get better, won't he?' cannot be answered 'yes' because nobody knows. You can be truthful without building up too much hope by saying that the longer the heart can be controlled and rested, and provided no complications arise, the greater the chances of recovery. The fact that the relative has posed the question demonstrates that there is doubt in her or his mind. Offer to discuss further care and practical ways of helping the patient when the condition has improved, but the doctor may like to see the relative immediately. It is useful to be present during the interview with the doctor so that you (or Sister) are sure you understand what has been said. In states of anxiety relatives cannot remember what was said and confuse words and understanding. Keep any instructions to the relative simple and write down telephone numbers, ward name, etc. If possible the relative may wish to stay. Care of the relative is as important as care of the patient and often it is the nurse who has this responsibility. Allow the relative to cry. You don't need to talk – just be there and **listen**. A cup of tea often helps the relative to talk and relax tensions.

The nurse often has difficulty at times like this with her own emotions, but the touch of a hand can say a thousand words and it is not shameful for the nurse to show empathy. A caring nurse promotes relatives' confidence more than an aloof nurse, who may appear to lack feeling and understanding.

Patients suffering from myocardial infarction, hypertension (see Unit 5) or valvular heart disease are usually advised to:

1 Stop or reduce smoking (see page 17).
2 Reduce weight if necessary.
3 Exercise regularly (within personal limits), increasing as advised by doctor.
4 Reduce saturated (animal) fat intake.

For a quick and easy revision test on this unit, turn to page 111.

References

Boore, J. R. P., *Prescription for Recovery* (Churchill Livingstone, 1978)

Hayward, J., *Information a Prescription against Pain* (RCN, 1975)

Norton, D., McLaren, R. and Exton-Smith, A. N., *Investigation of Geriatric Nursing Problems in Hospital* (Churchill Livingstone, 1975)

Further reading

Ashworth, P. and Tarry, P. (editors), 'Breathing' (*Nursing*, series 1, no 6, all articles, September 1979)

Ashworth, P. and Tarry, P. (editors), 'Breathing' (*Nursing*, series 1, no 7, all articles, November 1979)

Durie, M. and Corrigan, A. (editors), 'Breathing' (*Nursing*, vol 2, no 27, all articles, July 1984)

Durie, M. and Corrigan, A. (editors), 'Breathing' (*Nursing*, vol 2, no 28, all articles, August 1984)

5 Care of the patient with altered blood pressure

5.1 The control of blood pressure

Maintenance of normal blood pressure is essential to maintain life, so that the blood can supply all of the body tissues with oxygen and nutrients. Any reduced blood supply or loss of blood pressure to the brain causes confusion and loss of consciousness. If this state extends longer than 3 minutes then brain death results. The kidney is another organ which is affected by hypotension, and acute renal failure may result.

Fig. 5.1 shows the body's normal responses which increase blood pressure. Knowledge of these responses is important when assessing any patient who has been shocked, or is in a state of shock. The urine output will be reduced. Any IV fluid administered needs careful regulation, because it is very easy to over-infuse the patient – see Unit 3 on fluid imbalance and central venous pressure.

Before considering the care of a shocked patient you need to consider how blood pressure is controlled.

The 'driving force' for blood around the body is the heart, which pumps blood out of the ventricles – approximately 70 ml of blood at each contraction. If you multiply this figure by the heart rate per minute it will give you the cardiac output per minute:

Cardiac output = volume per contraction × heart rate
i.e. Cardiac output = 70 × 72 = 5040 ml per minute.

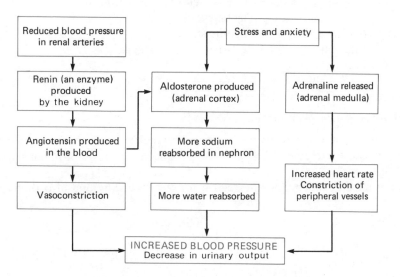

Fig. 5.1 The body's normal responses to hypotension (shock)

You can see that the heart, even at comparative rest, recycles a volume equal to the total blood volume each minute (in an adult). Exercise, anxiety or excitement will increase the heart rate and also the volume of blood ejected at each contraction. This increases the cardiac output in time of body need for oxygen up to a maximum of 15 litres per minute.

The next factor that influences the blood pressure is the size of the blood vessels. You do not have sufficient blood to fill all the blood vessels at any one time, so there is a system for regulating and redistributing the blood according to body need, e.g. to the muscles during activity; to the intestinal tract during and after a meal. Hormones, e.g. adrenaline, also affect the size of blood vessels, causing vasoconstriction to the peripheral vessels producing increased pallor. The control of vasoconstriction and vasodilation is illustrated in Fig. 5.2.

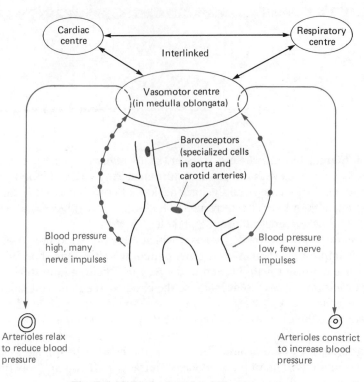

Fig. 5.2 Normal controls of blood pressure

Osmotic pressure due to plasma proteins also affects blood pressure (see Unit 3). In the following situations the blood pressure may be lowered:

1 Failure of the heart – cardiogenic shock.
2 Reduced blood volume – haemorrhagic shock (hypovolaemic shock).
3 Vasodilation of arterioles – anaphylactic shock.
4 Loss of control of the VMC – neurogenic shock.
5 Hypotension that cannot be elevated – irreversible shock.
6 Septicaemic shock.

5.2 Measurement of blood pressure (see Fig. 5.3)

Preparation of the patient is important

1 If the patient has never had his blood pressure recorded before, a simple explanation is necessary, because a degree of discomfort is produced – the lower arm feels tight below the cuff and the skin feels cold.
2 The patient should understand the reason for the recording and also the reason for the

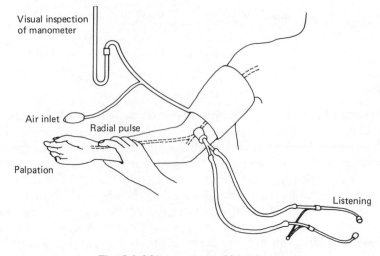

Fig. 5.3 Measurement of blood pressure

frequency, if taken on more than one occasion. Do not alarm the patient as this will raise the blood pressure.

3 The patient should be at rest for 10 minutes prior to the recording.

4 No tight clothing should restrict the arm or armpit, and the patient must be comfortable.

The equipment must be in good working order

Sphygmomanometer –	Check the cuff is the correct size. The width should equal two thirds length of upper arm. The length should firmly attach around the arm. The inflatable bag should not be perished.
Ensure easy inflation –	The valve in the cuff should be easily adjusted using finger tip control. The air inlet to the inflating balloon should be free of fluff and dust.
Stethoscope –	The diaphragm must be intact, and the ear pieces clean (danger of ear infections). The rubber tubing must not be perished.

Charts suitable for frequency of recordings are necessary.

Method of measuring blood pressure

1 Apply the cuff to the upper two thirds of the left arm – do not use an arm which has an intravenous infusion inserted. Place the manometer safely, at the same level as the cuff. The inflatable pad must be placed over the brachial artery.

2 Attach the cuff to the manometer.

3 Find the radial pulse and inflate the cuff until the radial pulse is occluded – note the level of mercury or pressure on the manometer dial.

4 Deflate the cuff completely.

5 Palpate the brachial pulse in the anti-cubital fossa. (This is medial to the mid-line when the hands are placed in the supine position and the arm is extended.)

6 Place the diaphragm of the stethoscope over the brachial pulse and re-inflate the cuff to a level approximately 10 mm Hg above the level of occlusion of the radial pulse.

7 Open the valve *slowly*, deflating the cuff. Note the level at which you first hear the brachial pulse – this is the SYSTOLIC pressure.

8 Continue to let the mercury fall, and note where the sounds change note or disappear. In some patients this may be simultaneous. The point at which the sounds change note is considered to be the DIASTOLIC pressure.

9 Chart the recording and remove the cuff.

10 Report any change from previous readings. If your reading differs from previous recordings, report your findings immediately to the nurse in charge. Your recording is most likely to be accurate, even if you feel inexperienced in taking and recording blood pressure.

11 Do not alarm your patient. Assess your patient generally
   – level of consciousness of the patient ⎤
   – any evidence of shock (hypotension) ⎬ make a rapid visual and
   – any headache (hypertension) ⎟ verbal assessment
   – respiratory rate ⎦

The recording you have made should be checked by a more senior member of staff.

5.3 Care of the patient in shock

The state of shock is a situation when the person is in a state of severe 'collapse', with pallor, cold sweating, absence of pulse or thin thready pulse, tachycardia and altered respirations. Anxiety levels are raised if the person is conscious, but often the person is in a diminished state of consciousness. The circulation of blood is altered causing a low blood pressure.

Fig. 5.4 shows the nurse's action for a collapsed patient.

The actual causes of shock are numerous, but they can be classified under five main headings. They are listed here with some causes.

1 Haemorrhagic/hypovolaemic shock – reduced blood volume and blood pressure falls.
   Causes:
   (a) Haemorrhage – usually more than 300 ml suddenly
   (b) Persistent diarrhoea – food poisoning or typhoid
   (c) Persistent vomiting – intestinal obstruction
   (d) Burns   **(e)** Excessive sweating – heat stroke
   (f) Excessive urine output
(b)–(f) are considered in Unit 3.

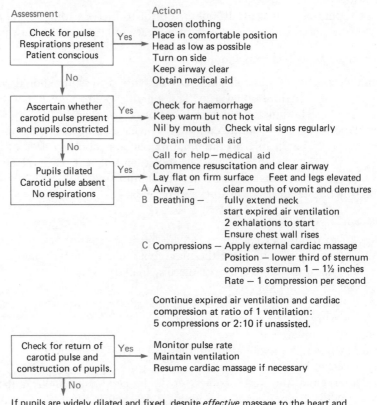

Assessment

Action

Check for pulse
Respirations present
Patient conscious

Yes →

Loosen clothing
Place in comfortable position
Head as low as possible
Turn on side
Keep airway clear
Obtain medical aid

↓ No

Ascertain whether
carotid pulse present
and pupils constricted

Yes →

Check for haemorrhage
Keep warm but not hot
Nil by mouth   Check vital signs regularly
Obtain medical aid

↓ No

Pupils dilated
Carotid pulse absent
No respirations

Yes →

Call for help—medical aid
Commence resuscitation and clear airway
Lay flat on firm surface   Feet and legs elevated
A Airway —   clear mouth of vomit and dentures
B Breathing —   fully extend neck
                   start expired air ventilation
                   2 exhalations to start
                   Ensure chest wall rises
C Compressions — Apply external cardiac massage
                   Position — lower third of sternum
                   compress sternum 1 — 1½ inches
                   Rate — 1 compression per second

Continue expired air ventilation and cardiac
compression at ratio of 1 ventilation:
5 compressions or 2:10 if unassisted.

Check for return of
carotid pulse and
construction of pupils.

Yes →

Monitor pulse rate
Maintain ventilation
Resume cardiac massage if necessary

↓ No

If pupils are widely dilated and fixed, despite *effective* massage to the heart and
ventilation of the lungs, within 3 minutes of the onset of cardiac arrest, then the
brain has usually suffered irreversible damage. The decision to cease resuscitation in
hospital situations is a medical decision, and therefore resuscitation should be
actively continued unless ordered to stop by medical staff.

Fig. 5.4 Assessment of the collapsed patient

2 Cardiogenic shock – reduced cardiac output, insufficient to maintain blood pressure. If the heart has ceased ventricular contractions, then a state of cardiac arrest exists.
   Causes:
   (a) Myocardial infarction
   (b) Acute left ventricular failure
   (c) Asphyxia, i.e. choking/drowning/road traffic accident
   (d) Severe respiratory disease of lung tissue
   (e) Pulmonary embolus
   (f) Overdosage of drugs that depress the heart activity or respiration
   (g) Paralysis of muscles of respiration
   (h) Cerebral disorder diminishing respiration
   (i) Electric shock
The heart depends upon its oxygen supply from the coronary arteries and any obstruction to this circulation, the oxygenation of the blood (via the lungs), or paralysis of the heart will produce cardiogenic shock and cardiac arrest if not corrected.

3 Anaphylactic shock – a massive vasodilation occurs of the body arterioles, often due to an antigen – antibody reaction, e.g. to X-ray dye, drugs, wasp or bee stings. Vasodilation causes a sudden drop in blood pressure, often referred to as a hypersensitivity reaction. **Causes** – this may be caused by many substances in sufficient quantities in susceptible people. It is of vital importance that the nurse ascertains any problems related to allergy:
   (a) Rashes, redness of the skin
   (b) Problems with certain foods
   (c) Problems with drugs, etc
   (d) Any history of hay fever, eczema, etc
These people should always have test patches or test doses of drugs and substances that are known to produce an allergic response, especially dyes, etc for intravenous programmes. Communication with the X-ray department is very important.

4 Neurogenic shock – the vasomotor centre which controls the normal blood pressure is overridden by the higher centres of the brain and the person may fall to the ground owing to pooling of blood in the peripheral parts of the body. This shock can occur with brain damage, following anaesthesia, or simply fainting. **Causes** – people often faint at the sight of blood, bad news or even sudden unexpected good news. Anxiety or tension will often exacerbate this situation.

5 Septicaemic shock – damage to capillaries results in blood and plasma in the tissues coupled with severe infection, e.g. peritonitis.

Not all patients who collapse have a cardiac arrest. Therefore, you should consider each main cause of shock, and the appropriate care required.(see Fig. 5.1).

FIRST AID for haemorrhagic shock

If the bleeding is arterial and external, i.e. being pumped out, and the blood is bright red:

1 Apply immediate pressure over the wound·with a clean cloth if possible.
2 Elevate the part if possible:
   (a) Nose bleed – sit the patient up if there is no alteration in the level of consciousness.
   (b) Arm or leg – elevate on a chair or nearby object.
3 Monitor pulse rate, respirations and level of consciousness.
4 Retain any articles containing blood to aid estimation of blood loss.
5 Promote relaxation of the patient by keeping calm and obtaining help quickly.

5.4 The patient with haematemesis (vomiting of blood)

1 Vomit may be of the appearance of coffee grounds, which indicates that the blood has been partially digested.
2 Vomit may contain large clots and frank blood which may have originated from oesophageal varices.

Care of the patient with haematemesis

1 Stay with patient and keep calm. Obtain medical and nursing assistance as quickly as possible.
2 Save all vomit in receiver, sheets, etc and quickly remove or cover soiled areas.
3 Lay the patient flat with one pillow in lateral position. Clean the face and provide a mouthwash. Monitor pulse and blood pressure.
4 Prepare for IV infusion/tranfusion. Nasogastric tube may be required. Morphine is often prescribed to assist relaxation of the patient.
5 Monitor pulse, blood pressure and respirations quarter hourly. Observe colour, evidence of restlessness, look for deep sighing respirations.
6 Follow medical instructions regarding nasogastric tube. Patient may have an emergency barium meal or gastroscopy.
7 Patient should have oral fluids withheld, unless the medical staff indicate otherwise.

If the patient is suspected of having ruptured oesophageal varices, a Sensgasten tube is passed into the oesophagus and inflated cuffs apply pressure over the bleeding vessel and hopefully stop the haemorrhage. The patient may have associated liver failure (see Unit 3).

The most common cause of haematemesis is peptic ulceration, which is usually treated conservatively with diet, and also with cimetidine which aids healing by controlling the production of hydrochloric acid from the stomach wall. It does not, however, affect the intrinsic factor so absorption of vitamin B_{12} is not prevented. Patients with peptic ulceration should be encouraged to:

1 Eat regularly and avoid heavily spiced food.
2 Take regular exercise and sleep.
3 Refrain from or reduce smoking.
4 Try to avoid stressful situations if possible on discharge from hospital.

Irritation of the stomach wall by drugs, e.g. aspirin, is another cause.

5.5 Nursing measures to ensure safe blood transfusion

1 Be aware of the complications of blood transfusion.
2 Ensure the correct patient receives the correct blood. Two people, one of whom should be

RGN, should read the labels carefully. Identify the patient by checking the wristband; calling the patient by name, if possible; checking the hospital number. Each unit of blood must be checked in this way at the bedside. Patients with the same surname must not be confused.

3 Blood administration should be commenced within 30 minutes at the most from the time of collection from the blood storage refrigerator. DO NOT STORE BLOOD IN THE WARD REFRIGERATOR. Blood cells start to deteriorate when exposed to room temperature for more than 2 hours.

4 Do not warm blood unless on medical instructions. Always use a blood warmer. Warming blood by any other means may destroy the blood cells.

5 Inspect the blood for discoloration and air bubbles. If these are present the blood must not be used.

6 Blood must always be transfused through a giving set with a blood filter. Blood stored in a blood bank does contain degradation debris, and this must be filtered out.

7 The siting of the infusion and commencement of fluid should be started using isotonic saline (0.9% normal saline) because this solution is compatible with blood. Dextrose 5% or lactate solutions should not be used.

8 The first 50 ml of blood of each unit should be delivered slowly to ensure no adverse reactions occur. Unless the patient requires blood very rapidly the rate of transfusion will depend upon:

    (a) Age of patient – elderly may have degree of heart failure.
    (b) Evidence of prolonged hypotension – may produce acute renal failure.
    (c) Liver disease may be present.

Each of these situations will require a slower rate of transfusion which will be prescribed by the doctor.

Care of a patient requiring a blood transfusion (see Fig. 5.5)

1 The patient should understand the need for the transfusion of blood. Information regarding any previous transfusion is necessary, particularly in females of child-bearing years. The blood group and rhesus factor are assessed by grouping and cross-matching the recipient's blood with that of the donor.

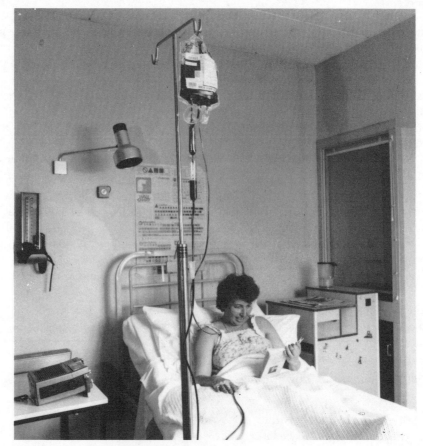

Fig. 5.5 Blood transfusion set

2 Prepare the patient by ensuring he is comfortable. The amount of mobility the patient is allowed during the transfusion depends very much on the reason for the transfusion. However, in the non-urgent, planned situation, the patient may be able to leave the bed for toilet purposes and sit in a chair as a change of position.

3 The siting of the cannula is the doctor's responsibility, but the nurse should assist, ensuring that the area has been shaved if hair is profuse, and that the bed area is protected. The patient's arm should not be constricted with tight clothing, and the transfusion bag must be able to pass through the sleeve of garments to facilitate changing of pyjamas, etc.

4 The patient should know how many units of blood are to be transfused, and when the transfusion should be completed. The limitations of movement should be clearly understood.

5 Support the arm (the non-dominant limb if possible) on a protected pillow, and instruct the patient to move the shoulder joint hourly. This prevents a 'frozen shoulder' which can be very painful, and results from immobility of the joint.

6 Observation of the patient and the transfusion is important.

  (a) Record temperature, pulse, respiration and blood pressure prior to commencing transfusion as baseline observations.

  (b) Record temperature, pulse and respiration frequently – according to local policy for the first hour of **each** unit of blood, and then hourly for the remaining blood. Report any changes.

  (c) Monitor the urinary output.

  (d) Observe for skin rashes, complaints of pain in back, headache, rigors, any rise in respiration or difficulty in breathing.

7 The blood should not be damaged by milking the tubing if the transfusion runs slowly. This damages the cells and releases potassium. If the transfusion needs to be speeded up, a pressure sleeve over the blood bag exerts a uniform pressure and increases the flow rate.

8 Observe the transfusion rate. An electronic monitoring device may assist the nurse to monitor the transfusion rate.

Calculation of flow rate

$$\text{Flow rate} = \frac{\text{Total volume transfused (ml)} \times \text{drop factor (drops/ml)}}{\text{Total transfusion time}}$$

Factors that can influence flow rate are:

  (a) Change of cannula position – bruising of tissues may occur.

  (b) The height of the transfusion bag is important.

  (c) Patency of the cannula – clotting may occur. Do not irrigate the cannula as the clot may be infected.

  (d) Venous spasm – a warm pack near the arm may reduce spasm.

  (e) Filter in giving set may be clogged. Infusion set or 'in line filter' may need changing.

9 Observation of the cannula site. 'OpSite', a transparent dressing, is ideal to enable observation of the cannula site. Any redness, swelling or bruising of the tissues should be reported immediately.

10 The giving set should be changed on completion of transfusion.

Complications of a blood transfusion

1 Circulatory overloading, which may precipitate heart failure

2 Allergic response – skin rash, elevated temperature

3 Reaction of mismatched blood: rigors, headache, back pain, blood in urine or diminished urinary output, chest pain

4 Pyrogenic reaction – blood may contain micro-organisms, material parasites, etc

5 Air embolism if air is allowed to enter into the tubing

6 Thrombophlebitis – an inflamed vein associated with clot formation. This is due to foreign substances irritating the vein:

  (a) plastic cannula

  (b) cannula not held firmly in position

  (c) infection entering at time of cannula insertion

  (d) irritant nature of infusion fluids which may be used

  (e) use of a vein for longer than 12 hours

7 Hyperkalaemia due to destruction of red blood cells:
   (a) nausea, intestinal colic, diarrhoea
   (b) vague muscular weakness
   (c) paraesthesia of hands, tongue, face
   (d) apprehension
   (e) slow pulse
   (f) flaccid paralysis
8 Hypocalcaemia – if a large volume of blood is transfused, sodium citrate is added to the blood to prevent it clotting. This substance prevents the calcium in the donor blood being available to the recipient. A low plasma calcium may result causing tetany.

5.6 Blood clotting

When bleeding occurs the blood clots in order to stem the flow. The clot has to be firm, and the blood loss, if severe, lowers the blood pressure, so reducing the possibility of the clot moving. Any patient who has been bleeding needs careful observation. As the blood pressure rises the clot may be dislodged and further bleeding occurs.

Mechanism of clotting – see Fig. 5.6.

Once formed the clot then retracts and pulls the edges of the torn vessel together.

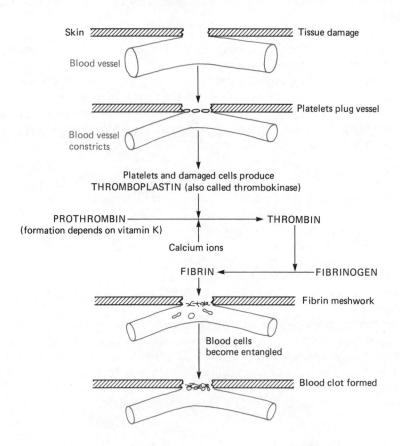

Fig. 5.6 The mechanism of blood clotting

Normal clotting time is 3–5 minutes.

Normal bleeding time is 2 minutes from capillary vessels.

Prothrombin time measures the activity of prothrombin in the blood. Prothrombin and fibrinogen are plasma proteins produced by the liver. Drugs (anticoagulants) may reduce the ability of the blood to clot:

1 **Warfarin** competes with vitamin K, and the liver takes up the warfarin in preference. Prothrombin production is reduced. The antidote for warfarin is vitamin K either intravenously or by intramuscular injection.
2 **Heparin** acts in several stages of the clotting mechanism, but mainly it inhibits fibrin formation. Heparin does not dissolve clots. The antidote for heparin is protamine sulphate by injection intravenously.

Thrombosis formation and embolism

Any factors that are likely to increase damage to blood vessels and platelets will increase the incidence of the formation of blood clots (thrombi). These situations **in veins** are:

1 Venous stasis of blood – immobility.
2 Reduced blood flow (hypotension).
3 Dehydration – reduced blood volume.   4 Varicose veins – faulty valves.
5 Obstruction to flow – garters, etc; constipation; pelvic tumours.

In each of the categories above there are many causes, e.g. constipation and hypotension, and it is important that the nurse is constantly alert to the prevention of venous stasis of blood (causing deep vein thrombosis). A thrombus that is mobile becomes an embolus.

Thrombi can also occur **in arteries**, but are generally less common due to the increased pressure and rate of flow of blood in the vessels. The main cause of thrombus formation in arteries is atheroma, which are fatty deposits beneath the endothelial lining of the vessels (see Fig. 5.7). This causes narrowing of the lumen of the blood vessel and turbulence occurs. The turbulence increases atheroma deposition. Atheroma can break away and then become an embolism. Blood clots too are formed on the roughened surface of the vessel. These may move with the blood flow or occlude the artery.

Emboli can therefore be moving blood clots, moving fatty deposits or moving air – most commonly from IV infusions (see Unit 3).

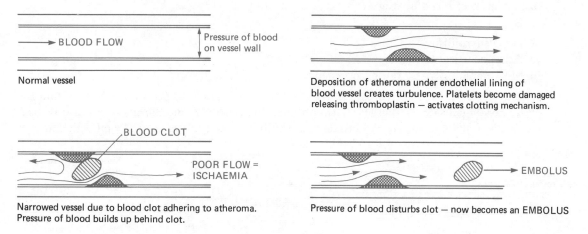

Fig. 5.7 Formation of atheroma

The care of a patient with pulmonary embolus (from a deep vein thrombosis)

The patient's problems will be:

1 Chest pain – sudden onset   2 Breathlessness, cyanosis, hypotension
3 Pallor, sweating – may lose consciousness   4 Extreme anxiety

Nursing care should include:

1 Stay with patient – monitor blood pressure, pulse, respiration
2 Obtain medical help
3 Administer oxygen – keep airway clear
4 Position according to the needs of the patient

Be prepared for the following:

1 IV infusion – 'life line' for drugs
2 ECG (electrocardiogram)
3 Chest X-ray
4 Anticoagulants – IV route then orally

Specific ongoing care:

1 Nurse patient at rest
2 Prevent further thrombus formation
3 Test urine daily for blood, observe for bruising
4 Report on sputum – amount and colour. Patient needs reassuring about blood-stained sputum

Health education:

1 Varicose veins – wear support hose
2 Advantages of exercise
3 Avoid standing for long periods
4 Rest with feet elevated
5 Avoid constipation

Advice if discharged on oral anticoagulants:

1 Always take prescribed dosage only
2 Do not take two doses together if one dose is 'missed'
3 Tick off doses on a calendar
4 Avoid fatty foods and oily aperients (inhibit absorption of drug), also alcohol and aspirin
5 Keep regular appointments at the clinic
6 Carry anticoagulant card ALWAYS – Inform dentist prior to treatment.
7 Remind doctor. Anticoagulants can be affected by many drugs.

5.7   Care of the patient with hypertension

Hypertension is usually said to exist when the diastolic pressure rises over 90–100 mm Hg, according to the age of the patient. Blood pressure tends to rise naturally as a result of increasing age and the arteries of the body hardening (arteriosclerosis).

Disturbances of blood pressure can occur as a result of:

1 Renal disease
2 Hyperthyroidism
3 Adrenocortical tumours
4 May temporarily rise during pregnancy

Raised blood pressure increases the work of the left ventricle to push the blood around the body. To compensate, it enlarges (left ventricular hypertrophy) and this may temporarily meet the needs of the circulation. Atheroma deposition increases in the arterial wall which further

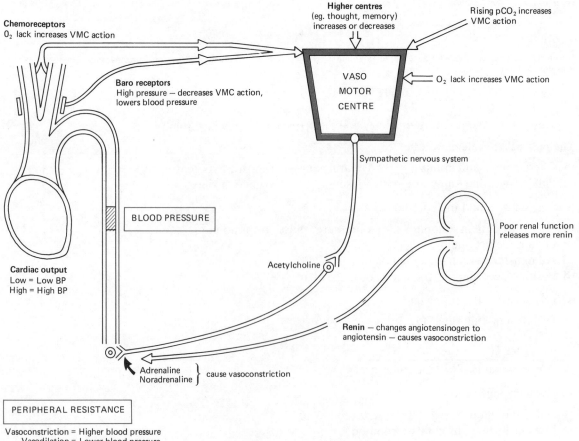

Fig. 5.8 Hypertension

decreases the overall lumen of blood vessels, so raising blood pressure. Fig. 5.8 shows the physiology of hypertension. **Other factors** that influence hypertension are:

1 Obesity   2 Smoking (causes vasoconstriction) (page 17)
3 Raised cholesterol from fatty diet – increases atheroma formation
4 Lack of exercise decreases utilization of body nutrients – increases weight
5 Stress raises blood lipids, increases vasoconstriction

Health education must include the need to:

1 Exercise safely   2 Reduce or stop smoking (page 17)
3 Reduce weight, if necessary
4 Try to reduce stress if possible

Complications of hypertension are increased by atheroma and are:

1 In cerebral arteries – headaches, cerebral hypoxia and stroke.
2 In mesenteric arteries – mesenteric thrombosis, gangrene of the bowel, perforation of the bowel.
3 In renal arteries – renal failure, increased hypertension.
4 In femoral arteries – arterial thrombosis, leg ulceration, gangrene and amputation of a limb.
5 In coronary arteries – myocardial infarction.

It can be seen that hypertension needs to be controlled, either as suggested by health educational measures, or by medication and relaxation. Atheroma increases clot formation and both atheroma and clots can break away and become emboli.

Assessment of the patient with hypertension

1 Any history in the family of hypertension should alert the nurse and the general practitioner to the need to monitor blood pressure regularly – hypertension is often discovered as a result of health insurance check-ups.
2 Headaches – assess frequency, position, intensity, visual disturbance.
3 Note any breathlessness or chest pain on exertion.
4 Volumes of paedal pulses in feet – are they equal?
5 Are there any mood changes or increased stresses?
6 Is the patient a smoker? Have they considered giving up the habit?
7 Assess patient's weight.
8 Assess diet, alcohol intake, if this is a suspected problem, and salt intake too.
9 Assess blood pressure after first ensuring rest and relaxation.
10 Test urine especially for specific gravity, albumin and blood.
11 ECG and X-ray will be required by the medical staff.
12 Tests of renal function, thyroid function and for phaeochromocytoma may be requested.

Care of the patient

1 Promotion of rest and relaxation is essential. This may be difficult to achieve. The patient may require a mild tranquillizing drug, and must be encouraged to talk through any problems or anxieties he or she may have. Help with relationships, finances, housing, etc may be required.
2 Measure and record blood pressure as required – e.g. daily, four hourly. May need to record pressure lying and standing with some forms of medication – postural drop. Be aware of the possibility of the patient fainting. Report any unsteadiness on standing.
3 Salt may be restricted in the diet, and this may be coupled with diuretics. These measures together with rest may correct the problems of hypertension.
4 Encourage the patient to stop smoking. It may be difficult and tact, diplomacy and understanding are needed when helping the patient. Why it is important to stop smoking must be clearly understood by the patient.
5 A reducing diet, low in saturated fats may be advised. The dietician should discuss the diet with both the patient and his or her spouse. Both of them may benefit.
6 Any headaches or altered behaviour must be reported immediately.
7 Medication should be taken regularly, and appointments for checking blood pressure must be attended.

8 Consideration of occupation may be needed. Can responsibility be shared or reduced? In this time of recession, pressures are often increased within the family and at work. Relaxation in the form of a hobby may be a valuable 'outlet'. Yoga and meditation may assist some people.

Activity

Look up drugs used to control hypertension. Do they act on the central nervous system, the heart or the blood vessels? What is the response to the sympathetic nervous system?

What are the side-effects of these drugs?

What does the patient need to know?

5.8   Care of the patient undergoing surgery

Shock is just one problem associated with surgery. The following care plans illustrate the case of the patient before, during and after planned surgery.

Preoperative nursing care plan

Problem	Aim	Nursing care
(Will be very variable according to individual) Patient very anxious. Not been in hospital before. Lack of understanding of what will happen and the nature of the impending surgery	Patient to understand the nature of the surgery	Accompany doctor when obtaining consent for and explaining operation. Return afterwards and ask patient to explain what he/she understands is to happen. Correct any misconceptions. Rephrase and reinforce crucial areas. Test urine and weigh patient.

	Patient knows and understands reasons for pre- and postoperative procedures
	    ECG
	    Chest X-rays
	    Special tests, etc.
		Explain all nursing procedures and reasons for the pre- and post-operative care and the patients role in these. Explain and show equipment in use after return to the ward. Spend time and allow patient to talk about operation fears and worries. Answer questions honestly.
		Understand the reason for preoperative investigations.

Removal from known companions and placed in stressful situation with unknown staff	Establish rapport and open communication between patient and staff	Ensure familiar nurse prepares, accompanies and collects patient from theatre whenever possible. Enquire whether visit from a minister of religion wanted. Be available to discuss problems. Explain any details again with patient and relatives. Encourage discussion with successful postoperative patients. Check patient's knowledge and understanding before preparation commences.
Anxiety due to loss of ability and loss of control over living activities	Patient will feel secure in the knowledge that his needs will be met	Allow patient to participate as much as possible in care planning. Check patient's satisfaction with care. Respect patient's wishes whenever possible. Maintain dignity at all times – avoid exposing patient and discuss matters quietly. Intimate tasks should be undertaken in a sensitive manner.
	Patient prepared physically for surgery as appropriate	Explain reasons for preparation. Patient to participate in preparation as required. Remove jewellery. Tape wedding ring.
	i.e. Clear bowel	Preparation may vary. Monitor effects of preparation, any results of clearance and report.
	Promote maximum cleanliness of skin	Preoperative bath/shower. Shave site if required. Care not to cut skin. Clean bed linen and theatre gown etc.
	Promote ventilation and aid expectoration if chest secretions present	Liase with physiotherapist – breathing exercises. Advise not to smoke. Promote coughing. Remove dentures. Prosthesese and nail varnish, etc.
	Prevent deep vein thrombosis	Instruct in plentar flexion/extension. Identify any circulatory problems especially varicose veins.

Potential problem	Aim	Nursing care
	Empty stomach	'NIL ORALLY' signs. Fast for 4–6 hours preoperatively. Remind not to eat or drink. Remove water and glass from locker. Check nil orally prior to leaving ward for theatre.
Fear of loss of security due to loss of control of the environment	Ensure the patient receives the correct operation and identity is clear	Premedication is given on time. Ensure identity band is securely fixed and details are correct and legible. Ensure consent form signed. Notes and X-rays available: any markings of operation site clearly visible and correctly marked. Registered nurse to recheck with patient.
	Ensure safety of patient on return to ward	Prepare bed when patient goes to theatre – clear locker. Bed in position for easy observation. Check oxygen and suction clean and functioning. Infusion stand. Charts correctly labelled. Vomit bowl/ tissues on locker.
	Ensure safety of patient in transit from theatre/ recovery to ward	Check operation site with recovery room staff. Instructions re drains, dressings are completed in notes. Doctors orders re fluid regime and analgesia is also written in notes. Ensure postoperative tray: oxygen and suction functioning on trolley, sphygmomanometer and stethoscope available if required.
	Maintain a clear airway	Place in semiprone position. Keep jaw forward and position tongue so that it is not obstructing the airway. Monitor respirations clear. Monitor colour, pulse rate, respiration rate.

Care plan for postoperative nursing

Problem	Aim	Nursing care
Patient has had surgery and is not fully conscious	To keep airway clear and promote ventilation of the lungs	Place in semiprone/lateral position. Airway remain *in situ* until removed by patient. Suction to remove secretion. Oxygen if required to increase oxygenation of the body tissue.
	Chest remains clear and free of secretions	Observe rate and rhythm of respiration ½ hourly. Monitor temperature. Reduce frequency of observations when stable. Sit up according to blood pressure and nature of surgery.
	Aid expectoration	Encourage coughing. Support wound. Encourage breathing exercises when fully conscious. Send sputum specimen for bacteriological test if necessary. Change sputum pot. Provide tissues and bag for disposal.
Pain of wound increased when coughing and moving in bed	Minimise pain to aid ventilation and promote mobility	Provide analgesia prior to chest physiotherapy and promote mobility. Report on effectiveness of analgesia.
	Maintain observations and to return to pre-operative baseline. Detect and report immediately any evidence of haemorrhage	Observe blood pressure and pulse ½–1 hourly to assess shock. Observe colouring of skin, pulse rate, sweating and skin temperature. Change position carefully. Check wound site and drainage – report. Repad if necessary. Empty, revacuum drains and chart amount and colour of drainage.
Dry mouth and possible feeling of nausea	Early recognition and treatment of fluid. Imbalance and paralytic ileus	Ensure infusion the prescribed rate and type of IV fluid. Record all fluid intake and output. Aspirate any NG tube. When bowel sounds heard, commence sips of water and increase fluid intake gradually to produce 1500–2000 ml urine daily. Report any nausea and vomiting. Provide vomit bowl.
	Promote rest and relaxation and prevent abdominal–bladder distension	Patient to pass urine within 10 hours. Change position 2 hourly. Check for bowel sounds. Pass flatus tube as necessary.

Care plan *(continued)*

Potential problem	Aim	Nursing care
		If patient catheterised – catheter toilet to minimise risk of infection. Closed drainage system.
	Promote wound healing. Early detection of any infection	Avoid any tension on wound. Leave dressing undisturbed if not contaminated. Aseptic procedure for redressing, shortening drains, suture removal. Monitor temperature 4 hourly. Investigate any increase in pain.
Mobility reduced. Confined to bed during early postoperative period	Prevention of complications of bedrest	Encourage leg and foot exercises and promote early mobilization. Avoid crossing legs. Use cradle. Check skin temperature in calf and assess if any pain or tenderness exists. Any preoperative problems with varicose veins may require TED stockings to be prescribed. Ensure they are properly worn and the correct size. Gradually mobilize to full activity.
Disturbance of normal eating pattern due to starvation	Introduce normal diet	When fluids tolerated well, commence easily digested diet and then normal diet. Add fibre to promote bowel action. Extra protein required to replace lost protein intake – aid healing.
Altered sleep pattern and increased need for rest	Promotion of rest and relaxation by promoting comfort – physically – emotionally – socially	Keep patient – family informed of progress. Answer questions openly. Maintain pain-free state by medication and good effective communication. Plan rest periods during the day. Night sedation if required. Observe for evidence of increased stresses. Assess the patients needs and prepare for planning discharge.
Inability to provide own personal hygiene due to effects of surgery and anaesthetic	Maintenance of normal level of personal hygiene Gradual return to independence in all activities of living	Keep skin cool and dry. Sponge hand and face. Change to own nightwear. Brush hair. Mouthwash after regaining consciousness. Return dentures. Early postoperative period patient may require a bed bath or assisted wash. Showering and bathing will depend upon the nature of the surgery and the former preoperative assessment of the patient. Particular attention to mouth care. Shaving the patient. (Some ladies too are embarrassed by facial hair.) Clean bed linen.

For a quick and easy revision test on this unit turn to page 112.

References

McMillan, E., 'Patient compliance with anti-hypertensive therapy' (*Nursing*, vol 2, no 26, June 1984), 761

Skeet, M., 'Saving Lives – First Aid in the Home' (*Nursing*, 1st series, no 14, June 1980)

Derrick Tovey, L. A., 'Complications of blood transfusion I' (*Nursing Times*, November 23rd 1978)

Derrick Tovey, L.A., 'Complications of blood transfusion II' (*Nursing Times*, November 30th 1978)

6 Care of the patient with elimination problems

6.1 Elimination

Elimination in this unit refers to the elimination of urine and faeces, and therefore revision of the following areas is important to facilitate understanding.

Activity

Revise

1 The gastro-intestinal tract – ileocaecal valve to anus.
2 The urinary system, including control of the bladder.
3 The muscles of the pelvic floor (see Fig. 6.1).

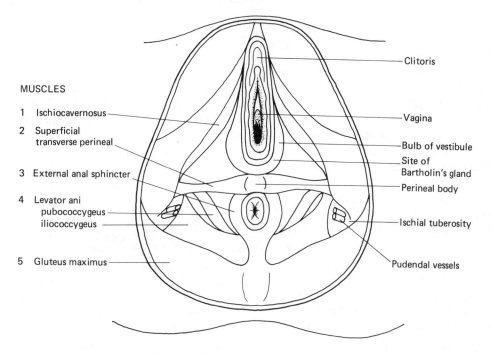

Fig. 6.1 The muscles of the perineum

6.2 Elimination of faeces

Elimination is a private function in the adult and a source of embarrassment if problems arise. Children at an early age learn to eliminate publicly and are given praise for the appropriate performance, and then gradually they are ushered to the bathroom, and public display of the genitals becomes unacceptable. The bathroom door is locked against intrusion.

All patients, on being ill, dread not being able to perform elimination functions in private. When there is an actual problem such as incontinence or the patient requires a stoma, this anxiety increases, and he or she may give up hope of ever leading a normal life again. Curtains round the bed do not overcome noise or odours. Embarrassment can cause problems of failure to empty the bladder and rectum.

Activity

Revise the structure of the colon, especially the muscle layer, blood supply and nerve supply.

The main functions of the colon are:

1 Absorption of fluid and electrolytes   2 Storage of formed faeces
3 Incubation of bacteria and synthesis of vitamins B and K
4 Propulsion of faeces towards the anus
5 Addition of lubricant (mucus) to the faeces

In order for normal defaecation to occur, the following conditions are necessary:

1 The gastro-intestinal tract must be intact and the muscles functioning.
2 The tract must receive a good blood and nerve supply.
3 The smooth muscles of the colon should respond to the stretch stimulus of the faecal mass, and the skeletal muscles of the abdominal and pelvic floor should contract normally to assist in the act of defaecation.

Defaecation is both an involuntary and a voluntary process. Faeces arriving in the rectum stimulate nerve endings in the rectum wall. Sensation is caused by the relaxation of the internal sphincter of the rectum, and the message is received via the enterogastric reflex of the autonomic nervous system. When the person is in a suitable environment for defaecation to occur, the external sphincter too relaxes by voluntary control, and the faeces are expelled.

If defaecation is not convenient the defaecation reflex will fade after a few minutes, to return a few hours later. Stored faeces may get hard and dry if this reflex is ignored too often. The person will then have difficulty with elimination (constipation) which may produce pain. Normally straining at stool should not need to occur as the stool should be smooth, formed and soft. Retrograde peristalsis will retain any faeces not expelled from the rectum into the descending colon. The rectum should, therefore, normally be empty.

Factors that affect bowel habit

1 Physical factors:
Congenital deformities of the bowel
Diverticulitis
Ulcerative colitis
Intestinal obstruction – volvulus; strangulated hernia; intussusception; paralytic ileus
Neurological lesions affecting the control of sphincters
Tumours of the bowel
Haemorrhoids; fistulas
Age (young and elderly)
2 Eating habits – type and quantity of food (see Unit 2).
3 Metabolic rate:
Reduced metabolic rate – myxoedema can produce constipation
Hyperthyroidism – patients may have an increased number of stools per day
4 Drugs:
Morphine, pethidine and codeine, reduce bowel propulsion and produce constipation
Antibiotics – may produce diarrhoea
Magnesium trisilicate taken in excess can produce diarrhoea
These are only a few examples of different groups of drugs

5 Emotional state. Anxiety increases reflex action and increases colonic activity. This produces frequent loose stools – diarrhoea. Continuous worry or stress may increase 'mixing movements' of colon and more water is absorbed producing pain or cramp at the sigmoid colon – irritable bowel syndrome.

6.3   Care of the patient with constipation

Constipation is a common problem in the elderly, resulting in infrequent bowel action and hard stools which are difficult to pass. The result of this can lead to faecal impaction in the rectum. Mucus is increased and leaks from the anal sphincter as liquid faeces and the patient often complains of diarrhoea. Causes of the problems that lead to the problem of constipation may be:

1 Defective toilet habits, toilet may be outside or not easily available
2 Immobility due to arthritis or osteoarthritis, stroke or Parkinson's disease
3 Defective diet
4 Reduced enterogastric reflex results in failure to answer the call to defaecate
5 Diverticulitis from overstretched bowel
6 Emotional disturbance, depression, especially if living alone
7 Confusion

If a problem of constipation is identified in an elderly patient, the nurse must obtain a careful nursing history regarding bowel habits, facilities, diet, etc and medical staff should always perform a rectal examination.

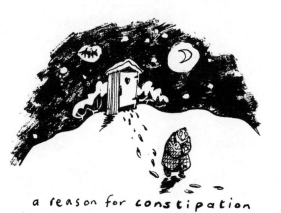

Fig. 6.2   a reason for constipation

Signs and symptoms of constipation often are:

Headache	Nausea
Anorexia	Loss of concentration
Halitosis and furred tongue	Depression
Flatulence	Insomnia
Irritability	Difficulty in emptying the bladder

Overcoming the problem of constipation requires:

1 Removal of the impacted faeces
2 Prevention of a reoccurrence of the problem
3 Ensuring that no existing bowel disease exists

If the faeces is hard and impacted in the rectum, it will require softening with a warmed olive oil retention enema, which may then be followed with an evacuent enema. 'Micralax' enema may be given but care is needed because hypotension may occur due to pressure changes in the pelvis.

Manual removal of faeces may be required if enemas are not successful. This is a very distressing procedure. The patient may require sedation. Manual removal of faeces should be undertaken by senior staff. The rectum could be perforated unless care is taken. Suppositories such as glycerine may be used to soften stools, or Dulcolax, which is a contact purgative, may be suitable if the faeces require extra propulsion out of the rectum.

When the rectum and descending colon have been cleared of faeces, oral preparations may be given and a high-fibre diet introduced. A stool chart should be commenced (see Appendix). Privacy should always be ensured during elimination and any discussion regarding bowel functions. Nurses often forget the indignity of asking an adult in the presence of others if they have had their bowels open.

Oral preparations that may be introduced are:

1 Faecal softeners – docusate sodium (Dioctyl)
2 Bulk purgatives – methyl cellulose (Celevac, Cellucon), bran, ispaghula (Isogel, Fybogel)
3 Osmotic purgatives – Epsom salts, milk of magnesia, lactulose (Duphalac)
4 Contact purgatives – bisacodyl (Dulcolax), senna (Senokot), cascara

Altered bowel habit, especially diarrhoea or faecal incontinence, should always be investigated because it may be due to bowel disease. Investigations that may be required if bowel disease is suspected are:

1 Sigmoidoscopy   2 Barium enema   3 Colonoscopy

All of these investigations must be preceded by clearing the bowel of all faeces.

Prevention of constipation:

1 Maximum exercise possible – if immobile the patient may be able to exercise the abdominal and pelvic floor muscles
2 Increase fluid intake
3 Promote regular bowel habits
4 Add fibre to diet to produce soft stools without causing diarrhoea
5 Provide alternative arrangements for toileting if facilities for elimination are inconvenient, e.g. commode if toilet outside

6.4 Care of the patient with diarrhoea

Any patient admitted to hospital with diarrhoea (often accompanied by vomiting) should be placed in a suitable position in the ward which is not going to cause the patient or other patients distress. Until the cause has been identified it is usual to adopt measures to prevent any spread of infection via the faecal–oral route – according to your local health district policy. Toilet facilities or a commode should be provided ensuring the privacy and dignity of the patient. THE PATIENT MUST HAVE THE FACILITY FOR HANDWASHING.

Activity

Causes of diarrhoea – how many can you identify?
Dietary causes   Drugs – groups of drugs
Disorders of gastro-intestinal tract – mechanical, inflammatory, idiopathic
Disorders of the liver   Disorders of the renal tract
Emotional disturbance   Disorders of the endocrine system

From your list you will see there are many more causes of diarrhoea.

Assessment of the problem of diarrhoea

1 General appearance of the patient – any evidence of marked weight loss, eyes, dry skin, etc.
   Look at the colour of the patient's skin – flushed, pale, grey?
   What is the texture of the patient's skin – dry/hot, cold/clammy?
   Do clothes fit loosely, is patient fully dressed?
   Any evidence of 'soiling'?
   Weigh patient and ascertain 'normal' weight if clothes were worn.
2 Behaviour of the patient:
   Is he mentally alert?
   Is he withdrawn, lacking energy, lethargic?
   Is he anxious, distressed, fidgety?
   Is he complaining of pain – knees drawn up? Pain continuing/colicky? – Is the problem impacted faeces in the rectum and faecal fluid leaking from anus?
   Are any drugs being taken at present time?
3 Observations of diarrhoea:
   (a) Advise the use of bedpan – provide facility.
   (b) Be sensitive to the patient's embarrassment and distress.
   (c) Keep your voice calm and quiet.
   (d) The patient must feel secure and wanted.
   (e) Explain any precautions if infection suspected.
   (f) Volume of diarrhoea – important to measure volume.
   (g) Note appearance – colour and consistency; blood – black, bright red; parasites present; undigested food; frothy.
   (h) Is excessive gas a problem?
   (i) Obtain specimen for medical staff.
   (j) Laboratory investigation – send immediately.
4 Provide vomit bowl and tissues, etc if required.
5 Assess appetite and food preference if the patient is able to eat and drink.
6 Are any social or emotional problems causing anxiety – this may be explored later during the patient's stay in hospital.

Activity

1 Look up your health district policy on its isolation procedures for various organisms, spread by the faecal–oral route.
2 Identify disinfectants and strengths recommended for cleaning toilets, crockery, etc.
   Policy related to handwashing, protection of uniform, etc, visitors. Do you **understand** this policy? Is it carried out correctly in wards?

If you have any difficulty, discuss the problems with your district officer responsible for control of infection, the ward sister or teaching staff.

Nursing care of the patient with diarrhoea

1 Keep the buttocks and anal area clean, and the use of a barrier cream will help prevent faeces causing excoriation.

2 A bath may be possible – be sure to clean the bath **thoroughly** after use with a cleansing agent which liberates chlorine, rinsing well after use.
3 Promotion of comfort is important, especially if patient is emaciated – use aids that spread pressure; turn two hourly (sheepskins may get soiled).
4 Keep patient warm but not hot. Sweating will increase the risk of breaking down tissue and normal fluid loss.
5 Maintain fluid intake to promote hydration, either by the oral or IV route.
6 Maintain nutritional intake, electrolyte intake and vitamin intake, as directed by medical staff. See Unit 2.

6.5 Care of the patient with a stoma

Stomas are formed often as a result of disease of the colon, e.g. ulcerative colitis, perforated diverticulum, tumour of the large bowel.

Stomas may be temporary, in order to rest the bowel, or permanent. Whatever the reason for the stoma, the patient requires careful preparation preoperatively and care and support postoperatively both in hospital and in the community.

As part of the preoperative preparation, the patient must know the reason for the planned stoma, and the advantages for having the surgery must be discussed. If preparation emphasizes an improved quality of life for the future, the patient is more likely to accept the stoma.

Advantages of having a stoma

1 Diet can usually be improved to enable the patient to eat a normal diet in the future.
2 Diarrhoea will not be a problem once the stoma has settled down after the initial surgery.
3 The patients' health will improve. They should become more active and can participate in sports, etc as normal. Special appliances are available for swimming, etc.
4 The complications of bowel disease are removed. These may be:
   Adhesions and fistula formation (in inflammatory bowel disease)
   Peritonitis from perforated bowel
   Anaemia from blood loss
   Spread of malignancy may be controlled and life expectancy increased
5 A stoma can be cleaned easily and can be seen to be clean. The anus cannot be seen and is presumed clean!
6 Less sickness is likely, which may improve chances of employment.

These advantages may not be possible without surgery. The disadvantages can be overcome by sensitive nursing care. How this is achieved will depend upon the preferences of the surgeon. It should be remembered that all rectal procedures to facilitate bowel clearance are debilitating and degrading, so privacy is essential, both of sound and vision. The patient may feel weak and depressed which increases the need for rest, sleep and emotional support.

Stoma site

This is important both for the patient and for the nursing staff. Medical staff should discuss with the patient where the stoma is to be placed. Appliances, seals and protection for the skin should be selected preoperatively according to the contours of the patient's abdomen. If appliances leak after surgery, the rejection of the stoma by the patient may be increased. The patient may like to wear the appliance preoperatively with water added to the bag. Often this increases the confidence of the patient. Fig. 6.3 shows possible stoma sites.

Assessment of the general physical state of the patient is important:

1 Full blood count – assess anaemia, hydration
2 Electrolytes and urea – electrolyte balance and elimination of waste by the kidneys
3 Group and cross-match blood – transfusion may be given preoperatively
4 ECG (electrocardiogram) – heart function
5 Chest X-ray
6 Body scan – if malignancy is the reason for the stoma
7 Body weight and nutritional assessment
8 Four hourly temperature, pulse and respiration
9 Ward urine test, especially for ketones
10 Assess the patient's susceptibility to pressure sores
11 Provide aids to prevent pressure sores

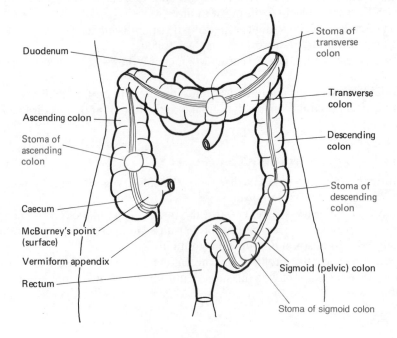

Fig. 6.3 Stoma sites

Care of the patient with a stoma will depend upon the actual surgery performed, but the following points are important:

1 The patient needs to accept the stoma as part of him/her self. In order to achieve this the patient needs to look at the stoma. This takes time, and the patient should not be forced. When cleaning the stoma ask the patient to hold a piece of tissue, or ask his or her opinion as to the cleanliness around the stoma. The patient may take a quick glance, and often the worst fears are not realized. The stoma becomes part of the patient.

Do not give it a name, because this encourages the idea of it being something different from 'self'. Gradually get the patient to undertake the care.

2 The patient must never feel dirty. Be careful about your facial expression. Never wear a mask or gloves, and use ordinary soap and water and toilet paper to clean the stoma. The use of a deodorant may help to reduce embarrassment, but let the patient have control. The spray, if required, is best used before the cleansing is commenced. Emphasize that a patient with a stoma is cleaner than a patient without one! The stoma, especially if a colostomy is in the descending colon, can be regulated as a normal bowel action. Ileostomies are more difficult because they produce faeces throughout the day, but substances that absorb water may make the faecal matter less fluid. A well-fitting appliance is essential in all cases.

3 The patient must have confidence in the appliance. The type of appliance must be acceptable to the patient and, therefore, the patient must be able to manage the removal and replacement of the appliance and any clip arrangement if a drainage bag is used. Patients with bifocal spectacles, arthritis in their hands or elderly patients require special consideration. The size of the appliance is crucial to the care of the skin around the stoma. The appliance should fit around the stoma leaving approximately a 3 mm gap between the appliance and the stoma. This applies to the application of Stomahesive or Karaya too. The patient should be tested for allergy to Karaya or adhesive used on bags preoperatively to avoid contact dermatitis occurring.

4 Disposal of the bags. Patients often refuse the offer of a special collection service by some local authorities because they feel 'labelled'.

The bag should be emptied down the toilet in the normal way. If the bag is placed inside a plastic bag and the top tied securely so that odour, flies, etc cannot cause a health hazard, the package can be concealed in a paper bag and placed in the dustbin, or burned in the garden rubbish. If out for the day, ladies may place the packet in the sanitary disposal bin or the container for paper hand tissues. Men may use this facility also. All that will be required to take out will be a small supply of tissues, a clean bag, and a plastic and a paper bag. These can easily be contained in the handbag or pocket.

5 Ability to play sports and to produce children should not alter in the female, although in men occasionally there may be a risk of impotence after surgery. During pregnancy, changing the appliance may become more difficult as vision of the stoma may be difficult. A mirror may be used to ensure the stoma is clean.

Care plan for patient undergoing colostomy

Problem	Aim	Nursing care
Normal pattern of elimination altered due to ostomy formation	Establishment of new routine Maintenance of optimum function	Observe colour, frequency and amount of faeces. Chart amount. If no action within postoperative 24 hours, check patency with gloved finger. Treat – irrigation/suppositories. After diet commenced, introduce foods and monitor effect. Involve dietician. Amend diet according to bowel action. Inform of foods likely to increase gas. If too fluid, increase bulk with cellulose. Advise eat slowly, avoid extremes of food temperature. Teach how to develop new routine, e.g. hot tea on rising to promote function.
Patient unable to care for ostomy due to postoperative debilitated state	Provide care for ostomy until patient is ready to learn	Treat aseptically until functioning. Check bag for action. Empty bag if drainable and chart/remove old bag and reapply bag. Measure stoma for correct size, repeating alternate days to ensure good fit. Observe colour of stoma daily.
Potential problem of skin excoriation	Maintenance of skin continuity	Clean site with soap and water and dry well. Remove traces of old plaster and secretions. Apply skin cream or protective barrier, e.g. Stomadhesive, Karaya seal. Stick bag firmly in place.
Potential problem of revulsion leading to rejection of stoma	Patient overcomes initial reaction and adapts to idea of stoma	Check patient's knowledge. Correct misconceptions. Educate regarding stoma and normal life style in future.
Possibility of patient behaving in aggressive manner towards staff, due to altered self-image	Patient works through aggression to accept stoma	Allow patient to express fears and negative feelings. Reinforce positive feelings. Answer all questions. Allow time to adapt to stoma. Encourage gradual involvement in care. Perform care to ostomy without fuss or distaste. Observe for signs of rejection and denial. If possible, encourage patient to examine equipment and wear a bag with warm water in it preoperatively. Arrange for a successsful stoma patient to visit and discuss problems. Encourage to join Ostomy Association.
Fear of rejection by loved ones due to presence of stoma	Patient feels secure in knowledge that loved ones will not reject him	Encourage verbalization of fear. Be available for discussion. Allow time and privacy for patient to express worries. Counsel relatives and explain patient's fears and situation. Support relatives in coming to terms with alteration in loved one. Encourage demonstrations of affection, touch, etc by relatives. Suggest psychosexual counselling if indicated.
Fear of odour and leakage	Ensure no odour and minimize leakage	Use odour-proof bags and air fresheners if needed. Check for good application of bags. Offer hospital clothing until action is predictable.
Lack of knowledge and skills needed to cope with ostomy	To teach patient to care for ostomy	Initially postop perform ostomy care and bag change for the patient. Assess patient's level of understanding and willingness to learn about ostomy. Plan teaching scheme on this information. Involve stoma care nurse, if available. Demonstrate whole procedure for patient. Break down skill into small tasks. Allow patient time to accept idea and then gradually take over care. Ensure equipment available for patient. Periodically check patient's progress.
Potential problem of stoma protrusion or collapse	Observation and early detection	Observe stoma daily for colour and size. Measure stoma alternate days to check size and for correct appliance.
Potential problem of wound infection	Wound heals without infection	Aseptic technique for dressing change. Observe for signs of inflammation daily. Record temperature four hourly at first.

6.6   The problem of urinary incontinence

Urinary incontinence is usually a more frequent problem than faecal incontinence and, therefore, often has a more profound effect upon a patient's life style. Before looking in detail at the problem, the normal bladder function must be considered.

Normal process of emptying the bladder

The bladder is composed of muscle, the detrusor muscle, and its function is to act as a reservoir for urine. In the detrusor muscle are stretch receptors which initiate the emptying process. The nervous control of the bladder is via the sacral outflow of the parasympathetic nerves and the lumbar outflow of the sympathetic nervous system.

In the child the bladder fills and in response to the stretch receptors being stimulated the spinal reflex causes the bladder to contract and the bladder empties. The adult normally has control over the bladder. When the nervous system is fully developed the central nervous system is able to control the reflex action of bladder emptying until the environment is suitable to facilitate relaxation of the bladder and urethral sphincter. Strokes or spinal injuries may interfere with this overriding control of the bladder and the patient may become incontinent. The muscles of the pelvic floor are important when considering control of the bladder. They assist in keeping the pelvic organs in position, which include the bladder. In the female, the pelvic floor muscles may be stretched owing to repeated pregnancy. Coughing, sneezing, laughing, running for the bus, etc may produce increased pressure inside the bladder and the sphincters become unable to control urine loss.

Many women may accept this as a process of life, and do nothing about it. They are embarrassed and in order to prevent 'accidents' may lead a life centred around the home or local shops only. Body odour may be a problem in warm weather especially even in the most scrupulously clean person. Urinary infections too may bring added distress, because the bladder may not empty completely and stasis of urine occurs.

Males have different problems often due to retention of urine. The prostate gland normally becomes enlarged with advancing age, and this interferes with bladder emptying. Gradually the bladder is always full, and the overflow only is voided. This often causes dribbling incontinence, and the patient has difficulty in starting to pass urine, the stream is poor, and trousers and footwear are often soiled. Urinary infection is again a common problem.

Infection in the bladder is difficult to eradicate because of the difficulties with incontinence. The patient reduces his or her fluid intake and urinary infection increases. The infection can travel via the ureter to the kidney and pyelonephritis can result. Any infection of the kidney leads to destruction of the kidney tissue and renal failure can result from problems that have been in existence for many months or years.

Prevention is better than cure. Nurses have a special responsibility to prevent urinary infection especially if patients require catheterization. Often in midwifery, catheterization may be required, and strict aseptic techniques should be employed. If closed circuit drainage is employed catheter care and the type of appliance used are important to prevent infection.

Care of a patient requiring urinary drainage to prevent infection

These factors must be considered when preparing the equipment:

1 Choice of catheter   Size of the catheter
   How long is it likely to be required?
   Self-retaining/simple catheter
   Are specimens required? – sampling port
2 Choice of drainage bag
   Is the patient confined to bed, or could leg bags with extension kits for night be used?
   Is there a non-return valve in bag?
   Is there a drainage tap to minimize the need to disconnect from the catheter?
   Can the patient manage the appliance if going home with catheter drainage?
   In acute care, does the system have the facility for hourly urine totals?
   Bladder irrigation – the bag must be large enough to take urine and irrigation fluid.

The care of the patient must include the reason for catheterization. IT SHOULD BE A LAST RESORT IN CASES OF INCONTINENCE. Fluid intake should ensure a good urinary output of at least 1500 ml unless contra-indicated in areas of acute illness.

The promotion of continence

Assessment of continence

Before any treatment can be given, or nursing care designed to meet the need of the individual patient, an assessment of the problem must be made. Preferably the assessment should be in a

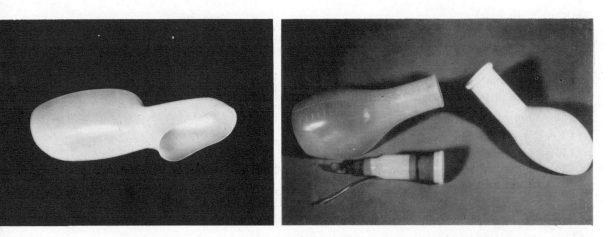

Fig. 6.4 Aids to urinary incontinence

private place, not in the ward with the curtains drawn. Often patients are deaf. Make sure that they are wearing their hearing aids if available. Questions should become part of the conversation, and should be designed to promote discussion.

Questions that may be asked:

1 How long have you been troubled in this way?
2 Did it start suddenly or gradually?
3 Do you have to get up at night? How often? For how long?
4 Do you have to go urgently? How much warning do you get?
5 Do you soil your clothes? Ascertain whether damp or wet.
6 Do you have difficulty starting to pass water?
7 Does your water burn or cause pain?
8 Does coughing or sneezing cause leakage?
9 Do you dribble after passing urine?

Factors that affect incontinence

1 Is there a pattern to the incontinence? Can a change in habit reduce incontinence?
2 Can the patient indicate the need to empty the bladder? (For instance, a stroke patient.)
3 Toilet facilities – distance; mobility of patient; upstairs or outside, etc; warmth and privacy.
4 Clothing; can it be adjusted easily?
5 Is the patient living alone? Depressed?
6 Is the patient confused?
7 Has the patient any constipation or gynaecological disorder?

Plan of care for the incontinent patient may include the following:

1 Patient will have a medical examination to establish any obstruction of bladder neck/urethra; disease of the bladder; disorder of the female reproduction tract; or constipation.
2 Keep a continence chart (see Appendix). Assess how long are the intervals during which the patient can remain continent. Provide facilities to enable bladder emptying before incontinence occurs. The patient should be near the toilet.
3 Maintain fluid intake to ensure good urine output.
4 Treat any urinary infection.
5 Provide exercises to the pelvic floor if the patient can co-operate.
6 Identify any cause for confusion if it exists.
7 Give praise for achievement.
8 Ensure privacy and dignity at all times.

If continence cannot be achieved, the use of aids, adaptation of clothing and appliances may help to reduce the problem.

Protective pads and pants are aids, and may give a patient added security and prevent embarrassment from dampened clothing. Further assessment is necessary before suitable aid can be selected for the patient:

What type of incontinence exists?
Volume of urine passed? Pads are variable in absorption rates.

Dexterity of patient?
Mobility of patient?
Sexual activity?
Mental state?
Is the aid available?
Can the aid be disposed of?   Other help available – can the spouse assist?

The patient must know how to use the aid:

> Change the pad when wet.
> Monitoring changes in pattern of incontinence.
> Clothing may require adaptation to prevent body odour. For dribbling incontinence, the pad should be changed two hourly.
>> Use barrier cream to protect the skin.   Wash after removing pads.

Incontinence requires discussion. It must be seen in relation to the entire emotional, social, and physical well being and self-esteem of the patient.

Activity

Identify the different types of incontinence aids available in your health department, and identify the following:

1 How much fluid do they absorb?
2 Are they suitable both for men and for women?
3 Are they usable if the patient is faecally incontinent as well?
4 Do pads come in different sizes?
5 What are the advantages/disadvantages of:
   (a) Plastic pants?   **(b)** Fabric pants?

Male collection devices

A disposable plastic penile sheath, which drains into a leg bag, is often very useful, and may be worn day or night.

Care of the skin beneath the sheath is important. A sheath which is too tight can cause pressure sores. Adhesive used to aid fixation must not produce an allergic reaction. Shaving the pubic area is advisable to prevent discomfort from adhesive tapes.

Female collection devices

With female patients, appliances are more difficult to design because of the anatomy of the genitalia. Catheterization may have to be considered if the patient is ambulant; a leg bag should be worn. The patient must be able to manage the control of the drainage system, and easily be able to change the bag, minimizing the risk of urinary tract infection.

Services for the incontinent patient – a problem, not a disease

1 Medical services exist to identify causes – general practitioner, urologist, gynaecologist.

2 A continence adviser may be available. These are nurses specially trained to give advice and help a patient with the problem of incontinence. An important part of his or her role is to advise colleagues and other professionals on promoting continence, and advise on aids and appliances. They may be available in outpatient departments, health centres or make domiciliary visits in the home.

3 Continence clinics and advice from nurses, community nurses, health visitors and medical specialists will help.
4 Enuresis clinics – enuresis may the the result of an emotional upset, especially in children, or the child may be late in the development of the nervous system. Specialist advice, including a psychologist, is usually available.
5 Laundry service and collection – details are available in local health centres or GPs' surgeries.
6 Disposal of soiled pads – special collection by the local authority is available for incineration. Patients should wrap pads in newspaper and place in special sealed plastic bags or use a garden incinerator.
7 Aids centres – are usually in large towns and cities.
8 Red Cross – give a loan service of commodes, etc.
9 Pharmacy – stocks of aids will be ordered on request.
10 Health Education Council – leaflet available from health centres and libraries.

For a quick and easy revision test on this unit turn to page 113.

Further reading
Allen, S. and Brooks, S. L. (editors), 'Faecal elimination' (*Nursing*, vol 2, no 30, all articles, October 1984)
Blannin, J. and Goodinson, S. M., 'Urinary elimination' (*Nursing*, vol 2, no 29, all articles, September 1984)
Tierney, A. and Simpson, H. (editors), 'Faecal elimination' (*Nursing*, 1st series, no 17, all articles, September 1980)

7 Care of the patient with problems in temperature regulation

7.1 The control of temperature

The normal body temperature range is 36–37.8°C. Regulation of body temperature is essential for life. If we become too hot or too cold then our cells cannot function and we die. The body therefore has to be able to regulate heat gained and heat lost.

Heat gain

Keeping warm is one of our main preoccupations in winter, as we **gain** little heat from our environment. Fig. 7.1 shows the body's reaction to a drop in body temperature in order to restore it to normal.

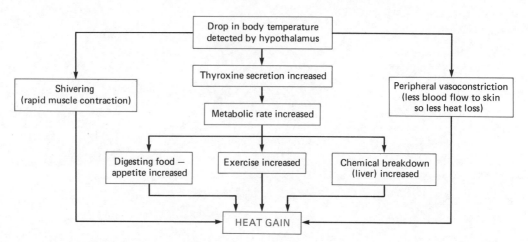

Fig. 7.1 The body's normal response to a drop in body temperature

Heat loss

Losing heat is important in hot weather. The body can regulate the amount of heat lost in several ways, as illustrated in Fig. 7.2.

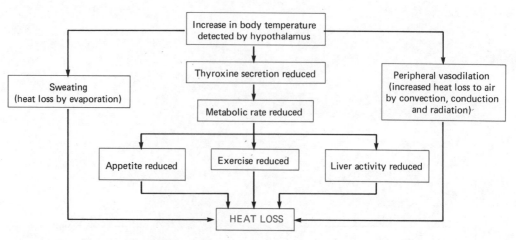

Fig. 7.2 The body's normal response to a rise in body temperature

The control centre for monitoring body temperature is in the hypothalamus. This links closely with the vasomotor centre of the medulla oblongata which regulates the dilatation of blood vessels to various parts of the body – especially the skin. The hypothalamus also links the body's entire nervous system, influencing sweat production (especially during anxiety and fear producing situations) and shivering.

The skin contains sweat glands all over the body, except for the lips, and the penis of the male. The sweat glands are most concentrated in the palms of the hands and the soles of the feet. We sweat constantly, though we may not be aware of the fact. Sweat production is increased if our body temperature rises, for instance during exercise, or if we have difficulty losing heat, for instance in hot weather. We also lose heat as water vapour from the lungs, and in urine and faeces.

The amount of heat lost from the body by convection, conduction and radiation depends on the temperature of the skin (i.e. the amount of blood beneath it), the type of clothing being worn and the temperature, humidity and movement of the air.

The surface area to volume ratio is greater for a small person than a large person. Therefore, a small person loses relatively more heat than a large person. A child, however, has a higher basal metabolic rate than an adult – a child is growing whereas an adult's body is concerned only with tissue repair. This explains why the elderly in particular have problems with hypothermia – they are smaller than a young adult but have a low basal metabolic rate.

Hormones are important in maintaining body temperature, especially thyroxine which regulates the basal metabolic rate. If too much thyroxine is produced, the body temperature may rise slightly, if too little, it may fall (myxoedema).

The temperature varies normally:

1 Between day and night.
2 At ovulation during the menstrual cycle.
3 An infant's temperature is higher than an elderly person's.
4 According to the position where the temperature is recorded (when the thermometer is kept in place for 2–3 minutes):
    Axilla – temperature lower than the mouth.
    Oral – temperature lower than the rectum.
    Rectum – temperature higher than the mouth or the axilla.

7.2 The pyrexial patient (see Fig. 7.3)

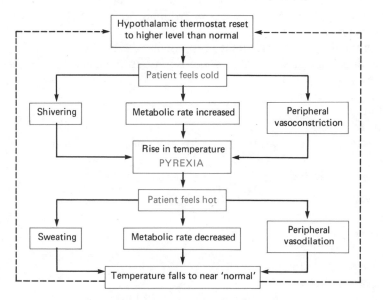

Fig. 7.3 Mechanism of pyrexia

Signs and symptoms of an elevated temperature are variable and may include the following:

1 General malaise, aching limbs
2 Headache
3 Cold, shivering, pallor
4 Hot, flushed appearance
5 Restlessness
6 Rapid respiration
7 Rapid pulse – may be full or weak
8 Dry mouth

  9 Profuse sweat
 10 Dry hot skin
 11 Delirium
 12 Loss of consciousness
 13 Convulsions

Causes of an elevated temperature

 1 Alteration of heat-regulating centre:
   Head injury
   Cerebral vascular accident
   Heat stroke
   Thyroid crisis
 2 Tissue destruction and inflammatory response – for example:
   Surgical interventions
   Peritonitis
   Injuries, road traffic accidents
   Myocardial infarction
   Damage to body tissues by excessive heat, corrosive chemicals, drugs, etc
   Tumour growth
 3 Invasion of the body by micro-organisms (bacteria and viruses) and protozoa (e.g. malarial parasites)
 4 Hypersensitivity reactions

Principles of care for a patient with pyrexia

 1 It is a medical emergency if the body temperature rises above 41°C. Always report any elevation in temperature.
 2 Monitor, record and report all vital body systems as appropriate.
 3 Adjust environmental temperature.
 4 Expose skin to air – cotton sheet.
 5 Increase evaporation of sweat – fans; cool by tepid sponging.
 6 Administer cool applications – ice packs in groin and axillae.
 7 Ensure complete bed rest.
 8 Give antipyretic drugs, e.g. aspirin as prescribed.
 9 Increase fluid and nutritional intake as appropriate to the cause of pyrexia.
10 Identify the cause of pyrexia:
   Complete body assessment
   Blood cultures
   Blood films (malaria)
11 Carry out appropriate medical treatment for any causative organism.

7.3   The hypothermic patient

Signs and symptoms of a lowered body temperature

 1 Slow pulse
 2 Slow respirations
 3 Shivering, shaking
 4 Cold pale skin, mottled in appearance
 5 Numbness of extremities
 6 Mental slowness, loss of consciousness

Care of a patient with hypothermia (often the elderly or very young)

 1 It may be a medical emergency if body temperature falls below 34.4°C. Monitor all vital body systems as appropriate.
 2 Conserve body heat – adjust environmental temperature. Room temperature to be about 28°C.
 3 Wrap patient in 'space blanket'. Monitor core body temperature.
 4 Monitor level of consciousness.
 5 If conscious give drinks at 37°C (normal body heat). Too rapid heating causes vasodilation and the blood pressure may fall rapidly, producing shock.
 6 Monitor production of urine (hypotension may produce renal failure).

7 Ascertain cause of hypothermia – social, emotional, physical causes.
8 Orientate the patient if confused.
9 Change position hourly. (There is a high risk from pressure sores.)

People especially at risk from hypothermia are the elderly, and contributory factors are:

1 The lonely and recently bereaved, depressed;
2 The elderly who have retired to the country – family not near;
3 The confused elderly;   **4** Patients with myxoedema;
5 The elderly with difficulty in mobility – shopping, etc;
6 Those with a limited income to cover heating, food bills, etc.

Elderly people are proud, and do not want to be a burden, so they struggle valiantly to keep up appearances of 'normality'. Supplementary benefits are available to assist in situations of financial difficulties, but often the elderly are not aware of them, or will refuse the money because it is considered 'charity'. Tact and diplomacy are necessary when assessing a patient's needs, and the medical social worker will be able to give detailed advice on these matters and the patient's situation.

Activity

Visit the DHSS. Find out the benefits available to the elderly (including pension). Assess the approximate cost of fuel, food and clothing for one month. What is your finding?

7.4 The body defence mechanism

The body has natural defence mechanisms and these include:

1 A healthy, intact skin enabling sensory perception so that pain can warn of damage – heat, cold, mechanical damage.
2 Hair, especially on the head, prevents heat loss, eyebrows divert sweat.
3 Mucous membranes – all body tracts that open to the exterior are constantly renewed.
4 The inflammatory system responds to injury.
5 The presence of some non-specific antibodies in the plasma.
6 The secondary defence mechanism (immune process) which is acquired and produces specific antibodies. This varies with age, the young and the elderly being the least able to resist infection.

Cells of the body involved in defence

The reticuloendothelial system is capable of producing cells able to phagocytize bacteria, viruses and other foreign matter, and also to produce immune bodies.

1 Reticular cells line blood vessels and lymph vessels and are found in bone marrow, spleen, liver and lymph nodes. These cells are often called 'fixed macrophages'.
2 Histiocytes are found in all body tissues and are similar to reticular cells. They can become mobile and are then called macrophages.

3 White blood cells (leucocytes) are mobile and protective, being transported in the blood. They can pass out of the circulation to the tissues. Normally there are 5000–10 000 mature leucocytes per cubic mm of blood. Some cells contain granules in their cytoplasm and are collectively called granulocytes. These cells are found and stored in the bone marrow. Other white cells have clear cytoplasm, and these are formed mainly in the lymph glands.

Differentiation of white cells and their function

Granulocytes

Neutrophils 62.0% – phagocytize foreign matter
Basophils 0.4% – function unknown, liberate histamine when damaged ·
Eosinophils 2.3% – function unknown, become increased in hypersensitivity reactions and parasitic infections

Non-granulocytes

Monocytes 5.3% – capable of becoming large macrophages
Lymphocytes 30.0% – important in cellular immunity and tissue repair

Plasma cells are specialized cells found in the bone marrow and lymph nodes and are the primary source of circulating immunoglobulins (Ig's).

There are two main functions of the inflammatory response:

1 To destroy, neutralize or limit the effect of injurious agents
2 To assist in tissue repair

The inflammatory response

The injured cells release histamine, which is an immediate response to injury. Later substances called kinins extend the response. A momentary vasoconstriction is followed by vasodilation, which increases the blood supply to the area.

Capillaries in the injured area become permeable and plasma containing fibrinogen leaks into the tissues. This protein also pulls water into the tissues (osmosis) producing tissue oedema. The tissue fluid clots and fibrin forms a 'meshwork' around the area of injury and localizes the damage.

Neutrophils in the blood and histiocytes in the tissues invade the area and phagocytize injured cells and debris. Many substances, including bacteria, cause the release of a leucocyte releasing factor, which liberates thousands of white cells from the bone marrow so raising the white cell count. Lymphatic drainage increases and healing takes place when the inflammation subsides.

Activity

Explain how the cardinal signs and symptoms of inflammation occur, these being: (a) redness; (b) heat; (c) swelling; (d) pain; (e) loss of function.

Inflammatory responses vary in the type of exudate produced:

1 **Purulent exudate** (pus) contains dead or dying neutrophils (tissue cells). A common causative organism is staphylococcus. Abscesses may require surgical drainage. A tract from an abscess is called a sinus. A tract from the skin to another area, e.g. the intestine, is called a fistula. Sinuses and fistulae rarely heal of their own accord. A deep abscess may erode areas where infection can spread (generalized infection) or erode a major blood vessel (septicaemia, bacteraemia).

If no complications occur, healing takes place and scar tissue is formed.

2 **Serous exudate** is frequently caused by streptococcal infections. It often collects in serous cavities.
3 **Fibrinous exudate** is commonly produced by serous membranes, e.g. pleura, pericardium, peritoneum. Fibrin roughens the surface of the membrane causing friction and pain. Adhesions may occur between the layers of the membrane.
4 **Mucous exudate** from mucous membranes. Initially the exudate is 'thin' but it later thickens. If the exudate becomes infected it becomes mucopurulent.

If any infection cannot be contained at the site of infection, and enters the blood either directly via the blood circulation or indirectly via the lymphatic drainage, a state of septicaemia exists, and all body tissues are at risk. The release of protein that is not completely destroyed will cause malaise, headache and pyrexia. Large amounts of cortisol are released into the blood, which block the inflammatory process.

The inflammatory response is impaired when:

1 There is a decrease in mature white cells – leukopenia.
2 Agranulocytosis occurs (the reduction of granulocytes).
3 Neoplasm of bone marrow produces a large number of immature white cells and these cannot function properly (leukaemia).

When the white cell count falls below 1000 per cubic mm of blood, any infection is life threatening.

Activity

1 Identify the drugs which are called CYTOTOXIC DRUGS. What precautions must be taken by all nursing and medical staff when administering the drugs? Examine your district policy.
2 Identify common antibiotics and find out:
   (a) what organisms can they destroy and their normal dosages;
   (b) by what route they are excreted from the body;
   (c) what side-effects they may produce.

Micro-organisms may escape from the body from:

1 The respiratory tract;   2 The intestinal tract;
3 The genito-urinary tract;   4 Open lesions;
5 The blood via bites of insects, infected needles, etc.

Mode of transmission of organisms – remember micro-organisms cannot move of their own accord! They are transmitted:

1 By contact;
   directly with the source of infection;
   by indirect contact (fomites);
   by droplet spread;
2 By a vehicle:
   by food that is contaminated – food poisoning;
   by water, e.g. typhoid, shigellosis;
   by drugs, especially lotions and ophthalmic preparations if not packed for single use;
   by blood, e.g. hepatitis;
3 In the air:
   by dust, especially organisms which produce spores;
   as suspended evaporated droplets;.
4 By insects (e.g. the mosquito – malaria).

Factors that affect a person's susceptibility to infection are:

1 Age;
2 Reduced immunoglobulins causing absence or a lowering of resistance to a particular organism;
3 Reduction of white cells (leucopenia);
4 Presence of underlying disease;
5 Steroids, radiotherapy or antibiotics influencing the response to infection;
6 Virulence of organism and 'dosage' of organism;
7 Nutritional state of host;
8 Environmental conditions which may affect general health;
9 General emotional and mental state – any inability to cope with life, e.g. a depressive state, often lowers the resistance to infection.

Activity

1 Examine your local health district policy on the isolation procedure required to prevent the spread of infection. You will probably find the following classification, or a similar one:
   (a) Strict isolation
   (b) Respiratory isolation
   (c) Isolation of faecal–oral route
   (d) Skin wound – blood precautions
   (e) Protective isolation
2 Are these isolation methods carried out in the wards?
3 What are the implications to the domestic staff?
4 What authority does the ward sister have in her ward to ensure:
   (i) a high standard of ward cleanliness?
   (ii) the prevention of cross-infection by doctors, nurses and domestic staff?
5 What 'problems' have you experienced? How may they be overcome?

For a quick and easy revision test on this unit turn to page 114.

Further reading

Ayton, M. and Thornett, M., 'Infection' (*Nursing*, 1st series, no 29, all articles, September 1981)

Clifford, C. and Lascelles, I. (editors), 'Infection' (*Nursing*, vol 2, no 7, all articles, December 1982)

Clifford, C. and Lascelles, I. (editors), 'Infection' (*Nursing*, vol 2, no 8, all articles, December 1982)

Lockett, B., 'Post operative wound care' (*Nursing*, vol 2, no 11, March 1983), 309

8 Care of the patient in pain

8.1 Introduction

Pain is a complex reaction, not just the result of nerve signals to the brain from the site of injury. Patients undergoing the same operation experience a wide range of pain, from mild discomfort in one person to severe pain reported by another. Everybody has a pain threshold, but what is it that makes this threshold different in different people? There is no simple answer. Most of us have experienced pain that has led us to a visit to the doctor or dentist only to find that when we arrive at the surgery the pain has gone, or have felt ill at home by ourself only to perk up and feel well enough to go out when called upon by unexpected visitors.

One of the first pieces of research to be undertaken in this field was by Beecher in 1956. He found that soldiers who received their injuries during active service were much less likely to require analgesia than their counterparts who had received similar injuries in a road traffic accident.

Factors such as personality, cultural patterns, and social and educational background are also likely to affect a patient's response to pain.

8.2 Theories of pain

1 Specificity theory is based on the study of pain pathways. A painful stimulus excites nerve endings which carry the message to the brain as occurs for example when you cut your finger. This simple theory fails to take account of the many factors such as cultural that we have already mentioned. Fig. 8.1 revises the physiology of the sensory nerve tracts.

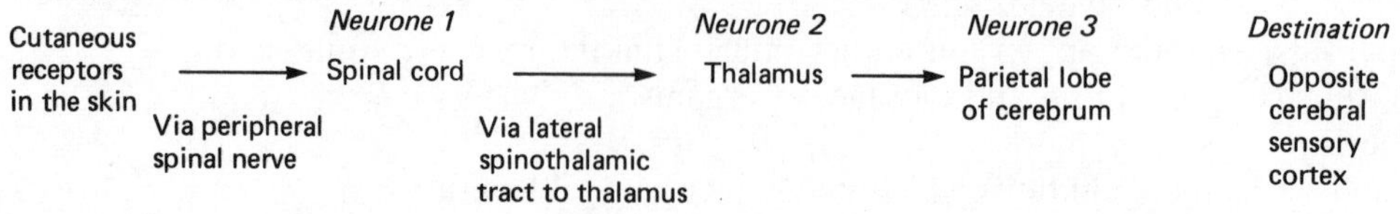

Fig. 8.1 Sensory nerve tracts

2 Pattern theory takes the specificity theory a step further. It recognizes that there are pain pathways but that these same pathways may also be used by other messages that stimulate the nerve endings. An example might be the sensation of being tickled. In response to the skin being stimulated in this way a person may respond with enjoyment or they may be annoyed and say that they are being hurt. This is a more complex theory and takes account of the fact that a person's state of mind influences his/her response to the stimulus.

3 Gate-control theory (see Fig. 8.2 overleaf) is the most complex of the three theories. It states that organized action of the body would be impossible if all the sensory input from the body were transmitted to the central nervous system, therefore the central nervous system must have a method of controlling sensory input. This control mechanism is referred to as the **gate** and is influenced both by internal and by external factors. This theory allows for the psychological and other factors mentioned that make a person particularly sensitive or otherwise to particular forms of stimulation.

None of these three theories is complete, but they serve to remind us of some factors that influence pain and its relief. Fig. 8.3 overleaf illustrates the various forms of analgesia.

8.3 Assessment of pain

Most would now agree that the only person qualified to know the level of pain the patient is experiencing is the patient himself. Somehow the patient through the limitation of language has to convey to others, at a time when his/her own defences are low, the extent and severity of his/her pain. To assist in this process various methods have been devised. The simplest of these is a preprinted list with various words describing the type of pain, for example a dull ache, cramp, stabbing pain, etc. A chart showing the body outline both front and back view is used in some units. The patient is asked to mark on the chart where the pain is felt. Rating scales may also be used to help the patient to identify the intensity of the pain. These scales may

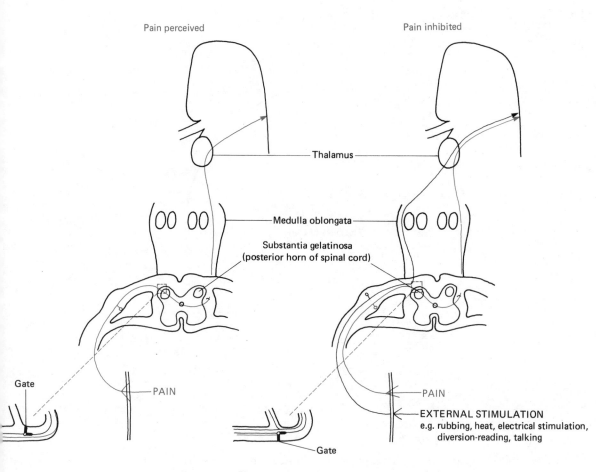

Pain perceived   Pain inhibited

Thalamus

Medulla oblongata

Substantia gelatinosa
(posterior horn of spinal cord)

Gate

PAIN   PAIN

EXTERNAL STIMULATION
e.g. rubbing, heat, electrical stimulation,
diversion-reading, talking

Gate

Fig. 8.2 The gate theory of pain

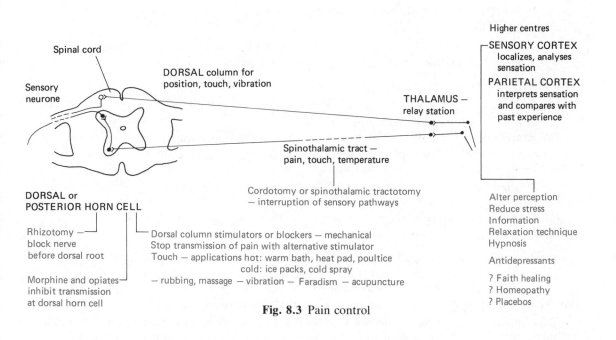

Higher centres

Spinal cord

Sensory
neurone

DORSAL column for
position, touch, vibration

SENSORY CORTEX
localizes, analyses
sensation

PARIETAL CORTEX
interprets sensation
and compares with
past experience

THALAMUS —
relay station

Spinothalamic tract —
pain, touch, temperature

DORSAL or
POSTERIOR HORN CELL

Cordotomy or spinothalamic tractotomy
— interruption of sensory pathways

Alter perception
Reduce stress
Information
Relaxation technique
Hypnosis

Rhizotomy —
block nerve
before dorsal root

Dorsal column stimulators or blockers — mechanical
Stop transmission of pain with alternative stimulator
Touch — applications hot: warm bath, heat pad, poultice
cold: ice packs, cold spray
— rubbing, massage — vibration — Faradism — acupuncture

Antidepressants

Morphine and opiates
inhibit transmission
at dorsal horn cell

? Faith healing
? Homeopathy
? Placebos

Fig. 8.3 Pain control

range from the simple three-point scale: no pain, moderate pain to intense pain to the more complex seven-point scale. See the Appendix for illustrations of the pain chart and the pain ruler.

Your own discrete observation of the patient is also very important in assessing the patient in pain. Many people do not like to complain and it is only when they are asked that their true state becomes apparent.

8.4 The cycle of pain (see Fig. 8.4)

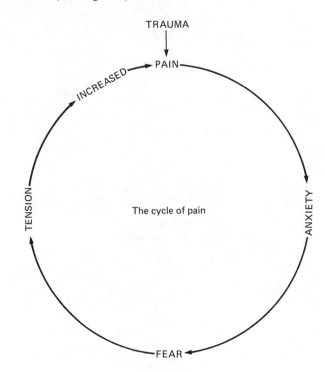

Fig. 8.4 The cycle of pain

Breaking into the cycle of pain

1 Relieve the cause of injury – set the broken bone; remove the irritant that caused the inflammation; remove the abscess that caused the pressure. These methods are based on the theory of specificity and generally invoke medical treatment. These measures will give a degree of immediate relief.

2 Remove the anxiety – keep the patient informed; build up a state of trust; ensure presence of a person who can empathize; avoid letting the patient feel isolated, angry, frustrated or frightened. These methods are based on the theory of gate-control.

3 Give appropriate relief – This could include any of the following: ice packs, poultices, hot water bottles, inhalations, massage with or without a liniment and drugs.

Analgesics (drugs to relieve pain)

1 Non-narcotics (many of which can be bought over the counter) include:
  (a) aspirin – very useful in rheumatoid disease
  (b) paracetamol (Panadol)   (c) codeine   (d) dextropropoxyphene
2 Narcotics or opiates (whose action depends on the release of the internal opiates, the endorphines) include:
  (a) morphine
  (b) pethidine
  (c) diamorphine (heroin)
  (d) methadone   (e) pentazocine

Narcotic drugs can cause the patient to become dependent upon them (drug addiction) so they are used with care, and largely in severe acute conditions rather than chronic ones. Thus for one of the arthritic type of diseases aspirin or paracetamol or a mixture of such drugs would be prescribed, changing drugs as and when necessary to gain maximum effect.

When pain is of a severe spasmodic nature, e.g. in renal colic, cholecystitis and labour, pethidine would be the drug of choice, because of its antispasmodic effects. Morphine or pentazocine are commonly used following major surgery for the first twenty-four hours. Diamorphine may be used in terminal illness.

In addition to these traditional forms of relief some units are using hypnosis, acupuncture and in midwifery, psychoprophylaxis with varying degrees of success in bringing pain relief.

It must be remembered that drugs must be given at the prescribed times if they are to have the maximum effect.

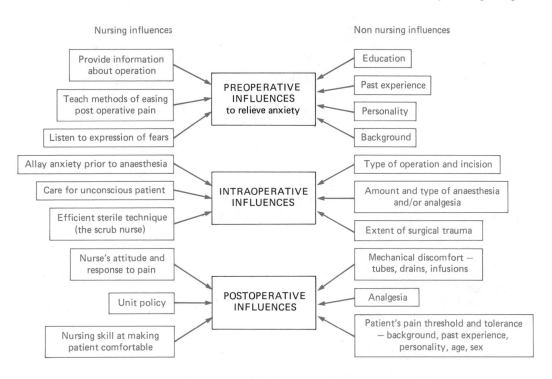

Fig. 8.5 Influences on the patient's perception and sensation
of pain following surgery

8.5 Surgical pain

Fig. 8.5 illustrates the factors which can influence the pain the patient perceives. There is a great deal that the nurse can do to alleviate postoperative pain.

8.6 Care of the patient in psychological pain

Psychological pain in this instance is not referring to pain that is not there, that is imagined, but to very real and often deep pain which is not the result of physical trauma. This is an area that since the Victorian era has been neglected in this country until fairly recently. To show no emotion was to be British. This attitude, however, does not stop the deep emotional hurt that is felt when a loved one dies. It may prevent talking about the pain but it does not make it go away. It is not just in bereavement that such pain can be felt, but when feeling misunderstood by friends, let down by the medical staff or when the nurse was rough and impatient today. The degree of pain felt and the reaction to it is going to depend on a multitude of factors. Some of these are discussed in Unit 11, where the whole subject is discussed in greater detail in relation to bereavement.

Care plan for the patient in pain

Problem	Aim	Nursing care
Patient perceives stimuli as painful leading to physical distress	Relief of distress by removal of stimuli, i.e. relieve pain. Early recognition and treatment of distress	Identify and eliminate source of pain if possible. Establish usual method of coping and adopt if possible. Administer analgesia promptly as ordered, before required. Observe the effects and side-effects, check with patient whether effect is satisfactory. Record and report effect to physicians. Monitor signs of stress: Pulse, blood pressure eight hourly; For facial signs, grimaces and teeth clenching; For restlessness and agitation. Plan care to follow after analgesia takes effect. Adopt other pain relief measures, e.g. relaxation, deep breathing, biofeedback. Apply heat – warm bath; or cold – ice pack, fan. Ensure open communication and allow the expression of feelings.
	Raise pain threshold by ensuring rest, relaxation and sleep	Plan rest periods during the day to follow analgesia administration. Plan care for when pain free – about one hour after analgesia. Lift and reposition carefully. Support limbs with pillows. Use pressure-relieving devices – sheepskin, bed cradle, light warm bedding or duvet. Position bed in quiet area of ward. Use night sedation when necessary. Use alcohol if helpful.

Care plan *(continued)*

Problem	Aim	Nursing care
	Alter perception of the stimuli by diversion of the focus of attention away from the pain	Provide company if required. Do not leave alone for long periods. Encourage to participate in care activities but without tiring. Encourage interesting activities. Provide magazines, jigsaws, radio, books, access to television. Liaise with occupational therapy. Encourage **short**, frequent visits. Encourage **brief** phone calls. Change patient's position regularly from bed to chair, position of chair, or to day room to chat with other patients.
Pain or fear of pain returning prevents or limits patient's ability to care for his own daily needs	Encourage participation in self-care activities as tolerated. Take over care if patient unable or unwilling to participate in self-care activities	Perform basic care activities in a caring and sensitive manner until patient fit to take over, e.g. bed bath or help to wash, sit up and clean teeth or offer mouthwash. Help change position.
	Symptomatic relief of problems likely to reduce pain threshold: Nausea/vomiting	Find out preferences. Provide light, nourishing meals often. Offer nourishing fluids – Complan/Build-up. Administer anti-emetics half an hour before food is offered. Use sherry to stimulate appetite.
	Diarrhoea/constipation	Monitor bowel function. Alter diet as necessary. Use bulk additives if indicated. Use two glycerin suppositories to soften stools.
	Cough/dyspnoea	Give steam inhalation four hourly; administer cough linctus. Sit upright. Order physiotherapy if helpful.
Potential problem of psychological stress, fear or anxiety due to pain and lack of ability to manage	Make pain easier to bear by provision of supportive environment which allows for vocalization of feelings, prevention or early recognition and treatment of psychological distress	Assess emotional response to pain. Explain effect of fear on pain. Establish open communications. Encourage discussion of feelings and **listen**. Allow demonstration of feelings, e.g. crying. Be available for discussion. Observe for signs of maladaptation, aggression, withdrawal, denial. Give prompt attention if summoned. Avoid false reassurances. Provide companionship if required. Support relatives where needed. Administer antidepressants if ordered. Involve clinical psychologist. Involve minister of religion if helpful.
Potential problem of patient feeling despair or helplessness and loss of control	Patient feels able to control destiny and maintain dignity	Involve patient in care planning. Ask patient to evaluate care. Encourage participation in care if possible. Inform patients **before** procedures. Respect patient's wishes where possible. Perform care activities patient cannot manage in a caring and sensitive manner. Do not rush patient. Do not ignore requests or isolate from conversations.

For a quick and easy revision test on this unit turn to page 115.

References

Beecher, H. K., *Measurement of Subjective Responses* (Oxford University Press, 1956)

Further Reading

Boore, J. R. P., *Prescription for Recovery* (Churchill Livingstone, 1978)
Blaylock, J., *Psychological and Cultural Influences on the Reaction to Pain* (*Nurses' Forum*, vol 7, 1968)
Hannington-Kiff, J. G., *Pain Relief* (Heinemann, 1975)
Hayward, J., *Information and Prescription against Pain* (RCN, 1975)
Hunt, J. *et al.*, *Patients with Protracted Pain* (*Journal of Medical Ethics*, vol 4, 1977)
McBride, M. A. B., *Nursing Approach, Pain and Relief* (*Nursing Research*, 16, 1967)
McCafferty, M., *Nursing Management of the Patient with Pain* (J. B. Lippincott and Company)
Melzack, R., *The Puzzle of Pain* (Penguin, 1973)

9 Care of the patient with mobility problems

9.1 Introduction

In this unit we will be considering the patients who, either in the relatively short term, e.g. the patient on traction, or in the long term, e.g. those with arthritis, have a problem with mobility. The very fact of not being able to get from A to B makes this patient totally dependent. What we need to consider are ways in which we can give these patients a feeling of well-being and what we can do as nurses to promote their independence. One of the common factors that may be limiting movement is that of pain. This subject is dealt with in a general context in Unit 8; therefore only the factors that are specific to this situation will be discussed here.

One major problem in losing mobility is the associated loss of independence. The following care plans detail the care of the partially dependent and dependent patient.

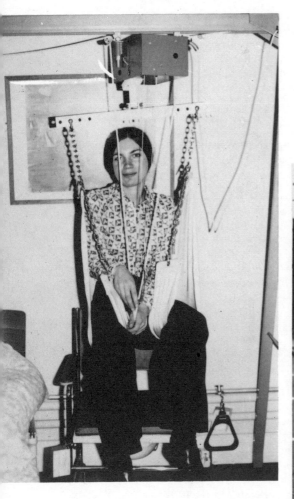
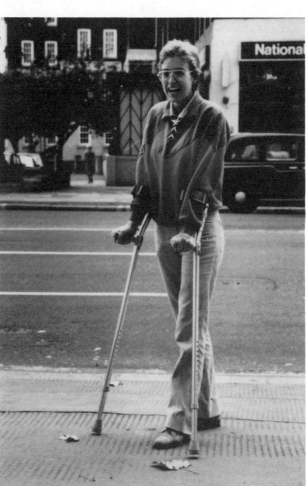

Fig. 9.1 Aids to mobility

Basic care plan for the needs of a partially dependent patient

Problem	Aim	Nursing care
Inability to perform usual hygiene functions unaided	Provide assistance to complement patient's limited ability – support those attempts to care for self	Offer bath or shower with assistance. Supervise patient during procedure. Organize equipment for bathing. Offer mouthwash and bowl. Help with feet and hairwashing if required. Assist with shaving if in difficulty.
Potential problem of skin breakdown.	Prevent skin breakdown	Encourage position change hourly to relieve pressure. Remind patient to move all limbs freely. Instruct not to cross legs in bed or chair. Ask patient to report soreness or numbness. Inspect at-risk areas while bathing.
Inability to move freely at will	Maximize independent movement. Assist, support where necessary. Use aids and prevent loss of muscle tone and function	Encourage active movement, or passive movements if impossible. Involve physiotherapist. Plan brief periods of activity. Help, support weight and allow to regain balance – use two nurses, then progress to one, then just stand beside in case of unsteadiness. Use wheelchair, Zimmer frame or walking stick to support weight.
Potential problem of falls owing to unsteadiness following a period of enforced immobility	Prevent harm to patient Maintain maximum muscle tone and balance	Provide support as appropriate. Check floors not wet and domestic appliance wires not across path. Check brakes on chairs and bed and rubbers on sticks. Check bath safety mat in use. Remind patient to use handles and use call bell if help required. Check footwear suitable – crêpe soles, clothing not trailing. Reassess skill regularly and amend plan as necessary. Do not restrict activities for safety reasons alone.
Difficulty with rest and sleep	Balance activity with rest.	Plan specific rest periods to follow activity. Monitor amount patient is doing and effect on level of tiredness.
Temptation to do too much and become overtired	Provide sufficient rest in day and sleep as near normal pattern as possible at night	Encourage gradual build-up of activity to tolerance. Make patient comfortable while resting in bed or chair with pillows, blankets, footstool or backrest. Promote more normal sleeping pattern. Offer milky drink or alcohol if not contraindicated.
Inability to maintain normal pattern of nutrition due to limitations of illness	Provide essential nutrients in manner suitable for utilization according to patient's limitations and preferences	Establish and maintain as near normal pattern as feasible. Ensure position most suitable for eating – sitting or side lying. Cut up food – ensure kept warm. Use spoon/fork, show special equipment. Assist when needed. If needed – pass nasogastric tube, check position, litmus paper (red), liquidize diet. Involve dietician, feed at correct temperature, keep nostrils clean. Or, if indicated, intravenous fluid, parenteral nutrition. Measure and record accurate intake. Observe for loss of skin-fold thickness. Provide hygiene measures before and after meals. If indicated ask relatives to bring in favourite food/snack. Ensure mouth and teeth clean and dentures in situ for meals. Use appetite stimulants, e.g. sherry, vitamin syrups. Remove difficulties if possible.
Inability to maintain normal pattern of elimination due to limitations of illness	Maintain or restore function, retrain normal habit	Establish and maintain as near normal pattern as possible. Ensure as near normal position as possible. Provide all necessary equipment in reach. Ensure maximum privacy. Use commode if possible. Answer requests for toileting promptly. Warm bedpan to 37°C with warm water. Offer facilities according to normal pattern. Provide washing facilities afterwards. Ensure fluid intake of 2 litres. Ensure sufficient fibre in diet. Monitor output of waste accurately. Keep stool chart (see Appendix) and send specimens.
Potential problem of urinary retention	Assistance if unable to eliminate urine independently – catheterize	Insert aseptically. Cleanse urethral orifice four hourly with soap and water. Fasten safely to leg to avoid pulling. Maintain closed system drainage. Observe output for abnormalities. Send off specimen if suspect infection. Ensure intake of 2 litres daily. If blocked – irrigate with half strength isotonic saline or sterile water. If leaking – change for smaller lumen. Administer medications to assist function, e.g. Cetiprin.

Basic care plan for needs of a fully dependent patient

Problem	Aim	Nursing care
Patient unable to meet own personal hygiene needs due to limitation of illness	Promote a normal level of personal cleanliness; ensure continuity of the skin	Daily bed bath – use own soap, flannel and towel if possible. Brush and tidy hair daily. Brush teeth three times daily, offer mouthwash. If cannot manage perform oral hygiene four hourly. Eyes – bathe with warm water twice daily. Nails – cut and file weekly. Involve chiropodist if nails hard. If required shave daily. Freshen hands, face and neck during the day.
Potential problem of pressure sores developing	Prevent or detect and treat sores quickly	Assess risk factor, e.g. Norton scale (see Appendix). Institute turning plan with chart. Turn two hourly. Observe sites at risk two hourly; if signs of redness turn one hourly and monitor. Keep skin clean and dry. Ensure careful lifting – no dragging. Ensure no crumbs or creases in linen. Use pressure-relieving devices – sheepskin, air ring, ripple mattress. Use bed cradle to relieve weight of covers. Prevent patient slipping down bed by use of footboard or sandbag.
Potential problem of chest infection due to stasis and pooling of secretions	Prevent, or detect chest infection quickly	Turn two hourly. Listen to breath sounds. Record respiratory rate four hourly. Record temperature four hourly. Involve physiotherapist in chest care, e.g. frappage. Use suction if cannot cough. Ensure fluid intake of 2 litres daily. Try to sit patient up and promote normal breathing and coughing. Send sputum specimen for analysis.
Potential problem of venous thrombosis due to poor circulation and limited mobility	Prevent thrombosis. Promote mobility	Encourage active movement through full range of each limb if possible – if not, perform passive exercises. Involve physiotherapist. Check no constrictions around calf. Check temperature and redness of calf four hourly. Instruct not to cross legs. Do not allow to sit with legs dangling while in chair. Use footstool, elevate end of bed.
Limited mobility, inability to change position at will – adapt a position of comfort due to illness	Provide mobility and position change for comfort. Prevent loss of joint mobility or contractures	Change position in bed one hourly; and from bed to chair. Maintain limbs in neutral position. Support with pillows, rings, sandbags. Relieve weight of bedclothes – use bed cradle or duvet and footboard. Involve physiotherapist for passive exercises. While caring for hygiene needs put limbs through full range of movement. Do not over-extend joints or strain muscles. Use pressure-relieving devices.
Danger of incidents or accidents due to inability to control movements	Keep patient safe from harm	Ensure limb alignment is correct. Lift and position in bed and chair carefully. Use brakes on both. Use cot sides. Use tip-back chair and tray. Check temperature of bath water and drinks. Place equipment out of harm's way. Check name band present, correct and legible. No smoking near oxygen points. Safe disposal of used materials, e.g. syringes. Ensure call bell available and working.
Potential problem of cross infection	Prevent cross infection from environment or other sites in body	Wash hands carefully before and after patient contact. Cleanse equipment carefully before and after use. Keep patient's belongings separate. Cleanse bedpans carefully after use. Use aseptic techniques.
Lack of ability to relax, rest and sleep – achieve comfort	Promote physical comfort. Relieve symptoms preventing rest and sleep: during day. at night. Promote psychological peace and comfort	Establish normal rest and sleep pattern. Try to maintain these if feasible. Plan set periods in the day for rests. Control noise, ventilation and temperature to make environment conducive to rest. Plan care together to avoid constant disturbances. Organize daily treatments and investigations to fit into routine if possible. Offer hot milky drinks or alcohol before bedtime. Administer night sedation if indicated. Ensure patient feels able to discuss important matters if wishes to. Explain how and why of nursing care. Provide emotional support to reduce fears. Be available for companionship if needed. Encourage visits by relatives or friends.
Potential problem of faecal retention	Prevent retention. Relieve – (i) soften stool and (ii) purgation. If fails, progress to more severe action	Try increased fluids and fibre first. Use two glycerine suppositories. Administer medication – Dulcolax or Senokot, disposable enema at 37°C. Use higher soap and water enema. Observe and report effects. Observe for side-effects – cramp, pain, wind.

Basic care plan *(continued)*

Problem	Aim	Nursing care
Stress, trauma due to social isolation from familiar environment and friends	Prevent or alleviate trauma due to isolation and provide meaningful relationships and secure environment within which open communication occurs	Provide companionship by establishing open two-way communication. Allow and encourage patient to voice their fears and anxieties. Be understanding and show empathy. Provide support and counsel when needed. Explain reasons for care planned. Involve patient in care decisions. Be flexible in routines. Enlist co-operation in care routines. Encourage visits from family/friends.
Potential problem of loss of ability to control own life leading to loss of morale and possible depression of mood	Patient must accept need for assistance and maintain a positive attitude to this need	Maximize independence in functions whenever possible or desirable. Involve patient in care planning especially short and long term aims. Follow his wishes whenever feasible. Explain when this is not possible. Involve patient in evaluation of care. Involve relatives in the care if desirable. Perform those tasks patient cannot manage in a caring and sensitive manner. Encourage vocalization and discussion of feelings. Review progress with patient regularly. Offer hope – if realistic. Keep informed about situation. Involve occupational therapist and minister of religion – if appropriate or helpful.

9.2 Care of the arthritic patient

To plan care for any individual, we need not only to listen and attempt to understand that individual, but also to have a knowledge of the underlying condition. The term 'arthritis' is a general one and is used to refer to two distinct diseases, osteo and rheumatoid arthritis, both of which will be revised.

Osteoarthritis

This is a common degenerative disorder affecting weight-bearing joints. It occurs in both sexes and symptoms first appear in the middle or later years of life. The main cause is probably wear and tear on the joints. Overweight, trauma and poor posture may be contributory factors.

Activity

Revise the anatomy of the skeleton (see Table 9.1).

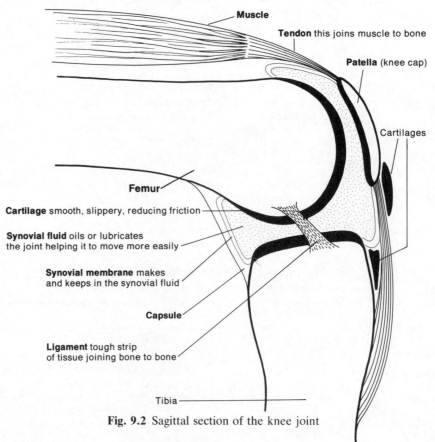

Joints are needed where two bones meet and will move against each other

Muscle

Tendon this joins muscle to bone

Patella (knee cap)

Cartilages

Femur

Cartilage smooth, slippery, reducing friction

Synovial fluid oils or lubricates the joint helping it to move more easily

Synovial membrane makes and keeps in the synovial fluid

Capsule

Ligament tough strip of tissue joining bone to bone

Tibia

Fig. 9.2 Sagittal section of the knee joint

Table 9.1 Revision of relevant anatomy and physiology

Part of joint	Function	Effect of disease
Cartilage	Shock absorber	Becomes thin and worn eventually wearing away altogether
Synovial capsule Synovial membrane	Keeps fluid in place Secretes synovial fluid	If ruptured loss of fluid and therefore inadequate lubrication
Synovial fluid	Reduces friction	
Ligament	Joins bones together	
Tendon	Joins muscle to bone thus allowing movement	Muscle spasm

In osteoarthritis bony outgrowths develop into the joint resulting in thickening of bone and protruding ridges and spurs.

Care plan for an osteoarthritic patient

Problem	Aim	Nursing care
Stiffness	Reduce strain on affected joint	Increase rest. Use mobility aids, e.g. walking stick.
Pain/limited movement	Reduce pain	Apply heat. Give aspirin/acetylsalicylic acid as prescribed. Reduce weight.
Muscle spasm	Relieve	Gentle exercise to maintain muscle tone. Encourage posture consciousness.

Other treatment

Many patients turn to osteopathy and chiropractics. Most of these practitioners practise holistic medicine and thus they can be very helpful in the early stages of this disease while patients are awaiting surgery. Their treatment will include advice on diet, including herbal remedies and teaching their clients good posture. They have time and usually build up good relationships with their clients. Their treatment improves muscle tone and can be very beneficial.

These days most patients eventually undergo successful replacement therapy such as hip or knee replacements. Where such replacement is not possible, care on discharge and follow-up will be similar to that for rheumatoid arthritis.

Rheumatoid arthritis

This is a very different disease, and one that forms a major health problem. It is a chronic inflammatory disease affecting connective tissue. In common with osteoarthritis it dominantly affects the joints, but can be further ranging. It results in crippling incapacity, affecting women three times more frequently than men. It can occur at any age, but more commonly in the 40s to 50s. It is thought that the disease is due to an autoimmune reaction because of the presence of the rheumatoid factor in 75% of the patients.

Inflammation and swelling of the synovial membrane and joint capsule result in granulation tissue forming. Fibrous scar tissue and adhesions develop. Calcification may occur. Treatment is directed towards the suppression of the inflammatory process, prevention of deformities and promotion of joint function.

Care plan for a patient with rheumatoid arthritis

Problem	Aim	Nursing care
General fatigue	Assess and alleviate fatigue	Rest. Carry out routine observations including temperature, as a low grade fever is often present. Take pulse rate – tachycardia is common. A full blood count will be taken as these patients are often anaemic.
Stiffness		Give heat and passive exercises; encourage movement.
Swollen, painful, red joints		During the acute inflammatory stage joints must be rested to minimize damage. Heat may be comforting. Splints may be used to maintain good positioning and to prevent deformities.

Care plan *(continued)*

Problem	Aim	Nursing care
Muscle weakness	Prevent atrophy	Encourage passive exercises and swimming which is excellent exercise for these patients.
Pain	Analgesia	Give aspirin regularly every four hours. Cortisone injections may be given into acutely inflamed joints.

Investigations

These would include blood for rheumatoid factor, erythrocyte sedimentation rate level (see Appendix), X-rays to assess joint damage, and assessment of limb movement and degree of disability.

Preparation for discharge

Has the patient stairs to climb – does he or she need re-housing in a ground floor flat or even sheltered accommodation? Are meals on wheels, or the home help service needed? Who will do the shopping? Will he/she qualify for a disability pension; invalid car or attendance allowance? Are appointments needed for:

outpatients; physiotherapy; occupational therapy; the day centre?
Is transport needed to get to these appointments? Do you need to organize transport?

Remember, the social worker needs to be contacted early as most of the services cannot be organized overnight. If a home assessment is necessary, remember to give the occupational therapist enough time to do this before the patient is discharged.

The nurse needs to ensure that the patient understands his or her condition so that he or she knows how to help themselves without causing further damage.

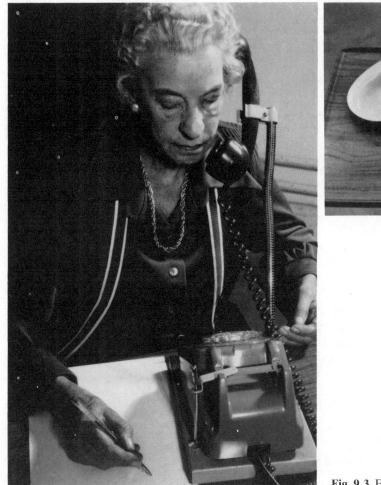
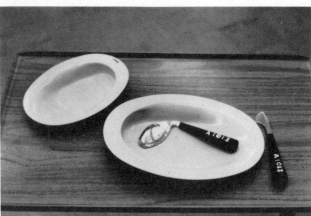

Fig. 9.3 Examples of aids available for the arthritic patient

Patients with this chronic disease and their families are faced with the added problems associated with a disease that waxes and wanes. In other words it is a disease that has periods of remission. Although remission gives a period of relief to all concerned, the return of the disease serves to dash hope and brings periods of depression. Physical or psychological stress appears to act as a trigger to the disease, which can cause a terrible strain on the family.

Members can suffer extreme guilt feelings if the disease reoccurs following an obvious 'family upset'.

This is a progressive disease with no real cure though occasionally the disease will 'burn itself out'. Diseased joints can be replaced which improves mobility but does not cure the disease. The drug treatment is drastic and can have unpleasant side-effects as for example with gold therapy or following a course of methotrexate.

Side-effects of gold

This is concentrated by the kidneys before they slowly excrete it, therefore damage to the kidneys can occur. The injections are cumulative so that at the end of the course the patient has a high gold reserve which can take up to 12 months to eliminate.

Other side-effects include: pruritis, dermatitis, glossitis, stomatitis, blood disorders, hepatic and renal damage. Serious side-effects are rare **if** the patient is carefully observed and the drug stopped at the earliest signs of toxicity. The urine must be examined for albumin before each injection.

Side-effects of methotrexate

This drug impairs the immune response so that it is more difficult for the patient to overcome a common infection. The bone marrow may also be depressed leading to anaemia.

It is therefore important to treat all infections promptly and to check the blood every two weeks for signs of anaemia.

Psychological factors

Most people know about the crippling side-effects of arthritis and so the pronouncement of this diagnosis is likely to produce an emotional reaction which the nurse must be prepared for.

Increased rest is usually necessary which, if the person works, can demand considerable reorganization of their daily routine. Social life can be considerably restricted which may lead to resentment not only on the part of the patient but also the partner.

Patients and their families often find tremendous support from their local ARC group and should be put in touch with them as early as possible. Sharing experiences helps both emotionally and practically.

The desperation of the disease has led many people to resort to unorthodox medicine. Many 'miracle cures' have been cited by people who have followed very rigid diet restrictions. It would appear that for some people hypersensitivity to certain foodstuffs causes the disease and to refrain from these elements in the diet brings about total relief from the disease. However, not all consultants hold with this method of treatment.

9.3   Care of the patient in traction

This patient can range in age from the toddler in gallows traction to the elderly. The range of conditions can be equally vast from fractures to slipped discs, with the traction being applied to the top or lower end of the body. Therefore, how can we discuss the needs of 'this patient'? The patient considered will be an adult, i.e. anyone between the ages of 18 to 50 years, with a

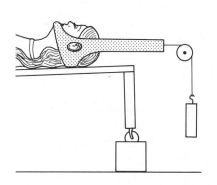
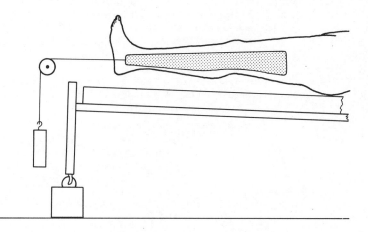

Fig. 9.4 Examples of traction

fracture of the lower limbs because it was felt that most problems of traction would be found here; the additional problems of immobility amongst the elderly are dealt with elsewhere. Thus for this patient we have the problems of the normally healthy, young, vigorous, active, independent adult strung up to their beds in forced confinement. The problems of the first weeks are often different from those of the long weeks that follow this initial period. Fig. 9.4 shows types of traction. See also the care plan for the patient with limited mobility (this unit).

The problems of boredom, frustration and isolation

After the initial period of not feeling well has passed these problems can lead to depression if not tackled. The following are suggestions only. The nurse and the patient are the only people who can solve the problem for the individual as so many factors will govern the course that is the most appropriate in each case, including the amount of activity and mobility that can be permitted without affecting the stability of the fracture.

The patients should be involved in all aspects of their care. Deep breathing exercises are essential if pulmonary complications are to be avoided. Active exercises of unaffected limbs including arms and shoulders are necessary to promote rehabilitation. They strengthen the limbs to enable them to take the extra weight and to use crutches once allowed up. The patients must be taught these exercises with full understanding of how to do them correctly – incorrect exercising could cause damage, therefore it is essential to supervise exercises to ensure the correct action and to encourage the patients.

Patients should be encouraged to remain part of the family; it is very easy to leave the absent member of the family out of decisions. Families need help in finding ways of including their hospitalized member. Patients may still be able to care for the financial arrangements, and continue to plan the meals, shopping and perhaps get ahead with the family's knitting requirements, darning and repairs that would normally be done at home.

Patients may use this time as an opportunity to continue their studies or to learn new skills. An imaginative ward sister permitted one of her active long-stay young patients to learn to play the guitar, an action that Tommy Steele has always been thankful for.

It could be an ideal opportunity for a person to learn new skills such as computer skills. However, patients will tire easily and a programme should be devised that will give frequent changes of activity, alternating exercises with periods of rest.

Once the traction is removed the patient is slowly rehabilitated. This can cause frustration as the patients can fondly imagine that once the traction is down they can get up and walk. The patients must therefore be given realistic expectations. Because of the prolonged bed rest and the elevation of the legs, the circulatory system needs to readjust or sudden elevation to the upright position could cause faintness. General weakness and joint instability is to be expected, but as activity increases, so also will confidence and strength.

Care plan for a patient with limited mobility

Problem	Aim	Nursing care
Limited mobility due to traction (e.g. fixed traction, Thomas splint)	Patient understands and accepts therapeutic need for immobilizing limb Provision of maximal mobility within limits of traction	Explain to patient function of traction. Inform of likely duration of traction. Demonstrate activities that do not interfere with traction and counter-traction. Rearrange furniture to ensure access. Provide monkey pole. Keep bedclothes light – sheets only. Encourage patient to alter position half hourly. Allow patient to care for his own needs as much as possible.
Potential problem of pain, discomfort and muscle spasm	Prevention or early detection and treatment	Ensure prescribed analgesics administered regularly as necessary. Ensure weights are not swinging, are fully suspended and nobody has moved them. Splints may cause pressure or friction. Check for infection at sites of entry and exit of pins. Ropes should be taut, riding freely over pulleys and free of bedding. Knots and adhesive tapes should be secure and not irritant. Bandages should be secure but not too tight. Limbs may be cold, discoloured, swollen or losing sensation. The under-sheet should be dry and free of creases and crumbs.
Potential problem of loss of muscle tone in unaffected limbs	Preservation of normal muscle tone and plan for rehabilitation	Refer to physiotherapist. Encourage isometric exercises two hourly. Develop upper limb muscles for crutches. Encourage good posture in bed.

Care plan (*continued*)

Problem	Aim	Nursing care
Potential problem of nerve damage due to pressure from traction	Preservation of nerve supply to limb	Check equipment daily or more often if patient complains of numbness or tingling in limbs. Check temperature of limb daily. Check correct space around top of splint, change if necessary. Check flannel slings daily – keep taut with no creases.
Potential problem of skin breakdown: around splint top; at heel; at sacral area and on elbows	Prevention of skin breakdown *or* early detection and treatment	Observe sites at risk four hourly at least. Keep skin clean and dry. Keep leather on ring soft by applying saddle soap or olive oil. Check sling tension and remove creases. Take care, lifting and moving, not to drag body. Encourage patient to lift self off sacral area. Provide air ring/sheepskin/ripple mattress. Keep elbows soft with cream and provide elbow pads.
Potential problem of deep venous thrombosis	Prevention or early detection and treatment	Check equipment daily. Ensure flannel slings and leg bandages correctly placed. Educate patient to report pain and heat in calf area. Encourage general mobility and deep breathing. Encourage patient to exercise toes half hourly.
Disruption and possible dependence in self-care activities, e.g. hygiene	Minimization of disruption	Provide all necessary equipment – bowl, hot water, mouthwash solution.
Disruption of normal pattern of ingestion and elimination due to limited mobility and awkward position	Minimization of disruption, and assistance when necessary	Ensure patient in best position possible for meals. Prop with pillows. Provide bed table at right height. Give light, nourishing meals – high in protein, vitamin C and calcium for tissue repair, high in roughage. Ensure patient understands need to drink 2 – 5 litres daily – prevention of renal calculi due to hypercalcaemia. Provide urinal/bedpan two hourly. Prop into most normal position. Provide privacy for elimination, use air freshener discreetly. Assess if problem with constipation: higher dietary fibre plus fluids; treat with stool softeners; suppositories or enema.
Potential psychological problems arising from limited mobility	Avoidance of problems: increase coping ability; provide support or help if necessary	Check patient understands treatment aim and duration. Discuss problems openly. Encourage maximum independence.
Potential problem of boredom or frustration due to social isolation and physical isolation from friends	Keep occupied and prevent problem of isolation	Position in ward near others in similar predicament. Arrange access to TV, radio, books, jigsaws. Encourage relatives/friends to visit and bring hobbies/crosswords. Develop meaningful relationship between staff and other patients. Provide possible diversional therapy, e.g. handicrafts.
Potential problem of economic worries due to lack of ability to work	Financial concerns minimized	Assess financial situation. Involve social worker. Provide sick notes. Contact employer if required. Involve disablement officer.

9.4 Care of the paralysed patient

Causes of paralysis include trauma; viral diseases; progressive diseases, e.g. muscular sclerosis; cerebral vascular accidents.

The care of the patient following trauma resulting in paralysis is a very specialized area and most hospitals would make every effort to transfer such patients to specialist units such as Stoke Mandeville. However, because of the nature of their disability they become fairly regular visitors to their local hospital, which is when you may first meet them. There are basically two golden rules to remember when caring for these patients:

1 The patient may be paralysed but that does not mean that he is 'stupid'. Many people, including unthinking nurses, direct questions to the accompanying relative rather than the patient. This does nothing to reinforce the patient's self-confidence or their confidence in the local hospital. It must be remembered that such patients have spent months if not years in specialist hospitals learning a high level of independence which has enabled them to return to the community from which you are now admitting them. The recent Olympic Games for the disabled showed that many manage to lead a more active life than those of us not so affected!

2 The patient will know more about his regular treatment than you. He knows what diet/appliances/aids work best for him. Respect his knowledge and encourage his continued self-care as far as possible. Do not try to persuade him to try different appliances; he has probably tried them all before and knows the disastrous results. There is nothing more demoralizing than a wet, dirty bed; you may not mind changing it, but it can rock the patient's self-confidence, and the knowledge that 'he told you so' may be of little comfort.

Progressive diseases

The patient whose injury is the result of trauma knows, once the phase of spinal shock has passed, the level of this disability and that it is highly unlikely that there will be any further improvement. Thus the long and slow adjustment to the condition can begin. However, patients with a progressive disease may never really know where they are. They may just be beginning to come to terms with being in a wheelchair when they have a remission and can once again be relatively mobile. The remission may last from weeks to years. When the remission passes and they find themselves immobile again it may come doubly hard as hope is yet again dashed. Like a child who is constantly teased, they are likely to be very angry and a tremendous level of understanding and patience is required. Patients and relatives need counselling support to enable them to come to terms with the condition, to help them all learn to live with uncertainty, taking one day at a time, for nobody can predict if and when another remission may occur.

The paralysed patients with whom you will come most frequently into contact are those who have had a cerebral vascular accident (CVA). They may be of any age, the younger age group commonly resulting from a bleed, the older group from a clot in the cerebral blood supply; in either case a degree of paralysis can result.

Rehabilitation

As soon as is possible one encourages a level of mobility. This has to be achieved gradually as the patient learns to, as it were, readjust to a 'one-sided' world. Thus the following may be considered as a 'typical' rehabilitation mobility programme.

Mobility – progress

From lying to sitting upright in bed;
From sitting up to sitting on the edge of the bed (this can take a lot of practice as the patient has to learn balance);
Transferring from the bed to the wheelchair;
Walking with the aid of parallel bars;
Ambulation using a walking frame;
Walking with a stick; and hopefully to walking unaided.

However, it must be remembered that the burden of carrying around extremities that may be dead weight requires tremendous energy expenditure. Therefore, patience and time are of the utmost importance in supervising the mobility programme. The patient should never be hurried or pushed beyond his endurance. An agitated patient performs badly and loses confidence.

It must also be remembered that these patients have a short attention span. It is therefore better to organize several short therapy sessions rather than one long one.

The patient who has had a cerebral vascular accident

It is recognized that the patient with a CVA may suffer problems other than mobility and these too are discussed, be it briefly. The patient under discussion will be past the immediate unconscious level as the nursing care of the unconscious patient is a subject in its own right.

Care plan for a patient with a cerebral vascular accident

Problem	Aim	Nursing care
Dysphagia (difficulty in swallowing)	Promote easy swallowing	Sit upright prior to meal times and for at least 30 minutes after food to facilitate digestion and to prevent aspiration of food. Give only small portions of food at a time. Turn head towards unaffected side to minimize dribbling. Press lightly on the right side of the neck when

Care plan *(continued)*

Problem	Aim	Nursing care
		food is in the mouth as this helps to stimulate swallowing. Place food in the unaffected side of the mouth. Allow the patients to feed themselves when and as able, starting with a small part of the meal. Make a list of the foods that the patient finds particularly difficult to swallow, so that these can be avoided. Have suction apparatus available in case of need. Provide mouth care after each meal.
Homonymous hemianopia (reduced field of vision)	Reduce distress, reorientate patient	Approach patient from unaffected side. Keep all necessary objects on unaffected side. Encourage patient to turn head to affected side frequently to help with their orientation.
Aphasia (inability to express oneself or understand speech)	Improve patient's communicative skills	Refer to, and liaise with, speech therapist. The patient's first attempts at speech may be 'automatic speech' which could include the use of swear words. Accept any attempt at speech and do not reprimand the patient for using 'bad' words. Although the answers that the patient gives may be unreliable, continue to ask questions because this encourages the patient to participate in the act of communication. Speak slowly and deliberately, facing the patient directly, and do not shout. Use gestures to reinforce verbal communication. While giving care talk about the patients' progress, their family, current events and other topics of interest to keep them aware of the social world of which they are part. Use pictures or flashcards as an adjunct to speech. Patients may point to one card when they really want something different; patience and understanding are paramount.
Poor memory	Promote understanding	This is both frustrating for the patients and the relatives and can outlast all other handicaps for these patients. For example once discharged they may be out shopping and forget what they came out for. Patients and relatives need to understand the long-term effects of stroke and to be patient with each other as they readjust to life together.

The greatest need of this patient is probably acceptance and understanding. Given time and encouragement many patients achieve a high level of independence. The nurse must resist the temptation to cope for the patient, and help the relatives to resist also. It may be quicker in the short term, but will not increase the patient's self-respect or facilitate his or her independence.

For a quick and easy revision test on this unit please turn to page 116.

Further reading

The Arthritis and Rheumatism Council, *Handbook for Patients* (ARC)
Disabled Living Foundation, *Kitchen Sense for Disabled or Elderly People* (Heinemann Medical Books, 1975)
Fallon, B., *So You're Paralysed* (Spinal Injuries Association, 1978)
Footts, S., *Handicapped at Home* (Design Council, 1979)
Guttmann, L., *Spinal Cord Injuries* (Blackwell Scientific Publications, 1976)
Hilt, N. E. and Cogburn, S. B., *Manual of Orthopaedics* (CV Mosby, 1979)
Joseph, M., *One Step at a Time* (Heinemann, 1976)
Powell, M., *Orthopaedic Nursing* (Churchill Livingstone, 1977)
Rogers, M.A., *Paraplegia: A Handbook of Practical Care and Advice* (Faber & Faber, 1978)

10 Care of the patient with altered body image

10.1 Introduction

This is a very personal subject and it may be difficult for us on the outside to understand what all the fuss is about in some situations. For example the distress of a pretty young girl who is severely disfigured down one side of her face and neck from extensive burns is understandable, but why should a middle-aged woman feel similarly following a mastectomy, or a young adult following colostomy? No one can see the results of the last two examples, whereas in the first example it would be difficult to hide the disfigurement from the world. However, the one thing that all the people listed have in common is that at some time in their lives they have had to come to terms with an 'altered body image'. For each of them it would have been a painful experience and the length of time taken and level of psychological adjustment that was achieved would depend in part on the level of support and understanding received from nursing staff, family, friends and fellow patients.

One way to help us understand what these patients are experiencing is to try to put ourselves in their shoes – how would we feel or cope? Do you have any scars on your body? I know several pretty young girls who refuse to wear a bikini because of appendix scars. If a young child points us out to its mother on the beach it reminds us of our 'incompleteness' which can be threatening and hurtful. Perhaps we should be unconcerned with what other people think or say, but our pride usually reacts. However, all of us would like to think that our body is perfect, the same as everybody else's.

It is not just children who are quick to pick out the abnormal, and the greater the abnormality, the more people will react. Take for example the young adult with severe spasticity. A very meaningful lesson can be had by taking such a person out for the day by oneself.

10.2 Care of the patient with burns

Caring for these patients is usually carried out in the regional specialist unit, so that few nurses in general training will meet severely burned patients. Thus a very general introduction to the subject will be found here.

The skin has five main functions:

1 Protection of internal organs from: injury; drying; infection.
2 Sensation: touch; pressure; pain; temperature.
3 Heat regulation via sweat glands and blood vessels.
4 Absorption – especially ultraviolet rays.
5 Storage of water and fat.

Fig. 10.1 overleaf shows the structure of the skin.

The assessment of the severity of a burn is made principally on the extent of body surface burned and depth of tissue damaged (see Unit 3).

Factors such as age, health and other injuries will also affect the seriousness of the condition but as a general rule of thumb if 10% or more of the body surface of a child or 15% of an adult is affected, the injury would be considered to be a major burn.

The depth of tissue damaged is classified by degrees:

1st degree – destruction of superficial layers of epidermis only.
2nd degree – destruction of several layers of skin, but sufficient dermal tissue remains to permit regeneration of the skin.
3rd degree – full destruction of the skin and some underlying tissue such as fat, muscle and even bone: granulation and scar tissue will eventually cover the affected area – skin grafting may be successful.

Generally young children and adults over 55 years have a relatively poor tolerance of burns.

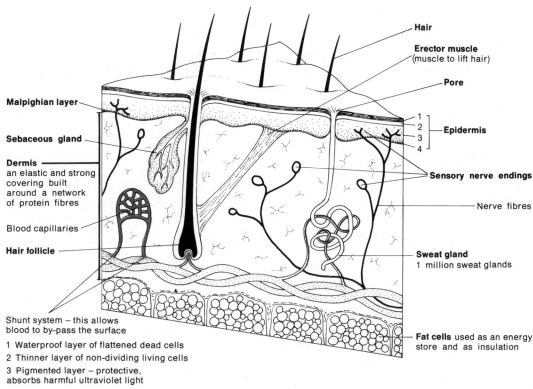

Hair

Erector muscle
(muscle to lift hair)

Pore

1
2
3
4
} **Epidermis**

Malpighian layer

Sebaceous gland

Dermis
an elastic and strong
covering built
around a network
of protein fibres

Blood capillaries

Hair follicle

Sensory nerve endings

Nerve fibres

Sweat gland
1 million sweat glands

Shunt system – this allows
blood to by-pass the surface

Fat cells used as an energy
store and as insulation

1 Waterproof layer of flattened dead cells
2 Thinner layer of non-dividing living cells
3 Pigmented layer – protective,
absorbs harmful ultraviolet light

4 Inner layer of dividing cells to replace those worn away

Fig. 10.1 The structure of the skin

Care plan for a patient with burns

Patient problem	Nursing care
Shock	This is the result of intense pain and fear. It can be so severe as to be irreversible. The doctor may give IV morphine and ask the nurse to monitor the patient's condition.
Loss of fluid, oedema and blisters	Increased permeability and dilatation of the capillaries results in a shift of protein-rich fluid which causes the blisters and oedema. This again is mainly a medical problem requiring a venous cutdown with plasma, whole blood and a plasma expander such as dextran being given. The nurse's role will be to observe the patient, particularly for signs of shock, blood reaction or cardiac embarrassment (see Units 2–4).
Hypotension	Blood pressure drops because of diminished blood volume and reduced cardiac output. May need to elevate the foot of the bed.
Wound infection	This can be the most serious complication causing death from septicaemia which may occur approximately 2 weeks after admission. Therefore, most units employ the system of reverse barrier nursing.
Contractures and deformities	Frequently check the alignment of limbs and body to prevent these occurring. Give passive/active exercises as appropriate to maintain joint and limb mobility.
Diet	This patient requires a high-calorie, high-protein, high-vitamin diet yet may not feel like eating. Ascertain favourite dishes and supplement with one of many preparations on the market (such as 'Build-up' or 'Complan') which will boost the nutritional intake.

Once the patient is over the initial period of shock the nurse needs to be on the alert for factors that may generate fear and anxiety:

1 Threat to life (e.g. infection of wound);
2 Permanent incapacity and disfigurement;
3 Prolonged period of dependence;
4 Separation from family and home;
5 Uncertain future;
6 Guilt regarding the accident.

Withdrawal, depression and resentment are commonly manifest. The nurse may help the patient through this difficult period by:

1 Being with the patient – so that he/she is not alone for long periods;
2 Encouraging the patient to talk through his/her fears and look realistically at the situation;
3 Involving the patient in occupational therapy;
4 Keeping the patient and family informed of progress;
5 Planning treatment together, particularly as this could involve prolonged reconstructive surgery and/or retraining for a more suitable job.

This patient is likely to experience difficulty in resuming social contacts. Patients and relatives need help in coming to terms with the new image. It may help if someone else, e.g. a nurse or counsellor, is present the first time the next of kin 'view the damage' if this has been kept covered. The shock the relative experiences can be reduced with careful preparation. This will include an explanation of the extent of the damage and a description of how it looks. A reminder that the person under the scar is the same person they married and still requires their love and support may help. The acceptance and recognition of the scarring by both partners is a big step forward towards social rehabilitation.

You are most likely to meet these people, not in the acute phase, but when they are admitted for an unrelated condition. Sensitive questioning is essential if you are not to alienate the patient. They may have come to terms, relatively speaking, with their new body image, but to give you all the details of the accident and subsequent rehabilitation may prove a traumatic experience as they find themselves reliving the weeks of pain and shock. If the patient shows signs of distress at your questions, change the topic. You may be able to gain the information you require from past notes, the admission letter or from a relative.

If the scarring is visible the patient may wish to wear a scarf or some other form of covering such as special make-up to hide the disfigurement. Respect this need and ensure that whatever they need for this purpose is always to hand.

Some patients may prefer to be nursed in a single room; if possible this should be respected. However, do ask and do not presume. The patient may not want to be shut away and may feel a social outcast if you place him or her in a single room.

10.3 Care of the patient undergoing amputation

The causes of amputation are:

1 Congenital;
2 Injury;
3 Neoplasm;
4 Peripheral vascular disease;
5 Diabetes;
6 Thermal injury – frost bite, burns.

Amputees broadly fall into two groups:

1 The elderly, for whom amputation, though traumatic as we will discuss later, results in an improvement of health – with less pain, increased mobility and therefore increased independence.
2 The relatively young. This group are likely to have suffered unexpected trauma, so that, far from bringing relief, amputation has a major impact both psychologically and socially.

There are in this country artificial limb and appliance centres, such as the one at Queen Mary's Hospital, Roehampton, where over the years specialists have researched into the best designs for prostheses, the type of operation and care of the stump postoperatively to ensure the best possible outcome. The nursing care discussed here, therefore, covers principles of care only. For the latest ideas in detailed care of the stump, write to the limb-fitting centre at Roehampton, or your own local centre.

If you are to nurse a patient who is to undergo an amputation you need to:

1 Make yourself aware of the level and type of amputation that is proposed so that you are able to teach the patient what to expect postoperatively and during rehabilitation.
2 Question patients carefully about their family, occupation and hobbies. This is essential in helping the team to plan and give priority to areas of rehabilitation: e.g. do they live alone? Have they stairs to climb? What type of work do they do? Will they need referring to the disablement resettlement officer? Will they need introducing to new hobbies?

One way of beginning to prepare patients psychologically for their new image is to explore with them what they expect of the surgery. If they see the amputation as, for example, a means of stopping the pain and increasing independence as they learn to walk, motivation is likely to be high, making rehabilitation a positive period. If, on the other hand, amputation follows unsuccessful attempts to save a traumatized limb, patients are likely to feel depressed and in low spirits. Such negative feelings, though totally understandable, do not make for good motivation in the initial stages of rehabilitation, which can prove a very stormy phase.

If possible a programme of exercises is taught preoperatively to begin to strengthen the muscles that will be needed with the prosthesis and for walking with crutches if it is a lower limb amputation. For the patient who will need crutches, success in their manipulation prior to surgery can prove a considerable encouragement.

The aim of surgery is to ensure a good stump. This is a stump that has sufficient skin and muscle, a good nerve and blood supply and a well-rounded bone end to enable the comfortable wearing and efficient working of a prosthesis.

Care plan for patient undergoing amputation

Problem	Nursing care
Immediate postoperative haemorrhage	Check dressing every half hour for first 4 hours then hourly for next 6–8 hours. Place tourniquet by bedside.
Swelling/oedema of stump	Firm bandages will have been applied in theatre which may need renewing.
If lower limb amputation	Raise foot of bed on blocks. Encourage to lie prone for 30 minutes three or four times daily to prevent hip flexion contractions. Encourage to move leg and stump at frequent intervals to improve the blood supply.
Pain	Needs sufficient analgesia to keep comfortable. Observe stump for signs of infection which must be treated promptly. Rewrap the stump bandage several times daily in figure-of-eight pattern. Must be firm to avoid oedema but at the same time must avoid stump constriction.
Phantom pain	The impression of pain in the amputated part of the limb is frequently present immediately after the operation but should quickly subside. If it persists this could indicate that the severed nerves in the stump have stuck to the scar tissue and further surgery may be necessary.
The stump	The attitude of the nurse dressing the stump will influence the patient's reaction to the new image. If she is repulsed by it and obviously dislikes dressing it, it will take the patient much longer to come to terms with the loss and slow down the process of rebuilding his/her self-image. The patient needs to learn to touch the stump and to come to terms with it as part of himself. The partner also needs to accept the new image and not be afraid of touching the stump.

Preparation for discharge may include:

1 Home visit to assess suitability to receive patient;
2 Teaching patient to:
    (a) Inspect stump daily using a mirror. Blisters, abrasions, swelling, redness, decreased sensation and other changes are to be reported to doctor.
    (b) Apply bandages if necessary.

Organize arrangements to continue rehabilitation programme as outpatient; appointments for outpatients' clinic; appointments for prothesis clinic.

10.4 Care of the patient undergoing mastectomy

Mastectomy used to be the routine surgical procedure for cancer of the breast. It was fairly drastic and very mutilating. Many women suffered severe psychological trauma following surgery. Would their husbands still love them now they were only 'half-a-woman'? Would he be so repulsed by the large ugly scar that he would never touch her again? Not only was the surgery drastic but the success rate was not too encouraging. Approximately 50% of patients diagnosed as having breast cancer die from the disease. However, it must be remembered the earlier the diagnosis the better the prognosis.

The breast is the most common site of cancer in the female, which occurs in 4% of adult women and accounts for approximately 20.7% of cancer deaths in Britain. Unfortunately, breast cancer readily metastasizes to the regional lymph nodes and other structures.

Breast cancer rarely occurs before the age of 25 years. The women that are particularly at risk of developing the disease are those whose close relatives, i.e. mothers, sisters, aunts and grandmothers, have suffered from breast cancer.

The patient and her partner need to be prepared for the altered body image following mastectomy. The patient may feel withdrawn, unresponsive or resentful that this should happen to her. She may feel helpless, lonely and abandoned. She will need the support of a nurse who is capable of understanding and accepting her feelings. The freedom to express her feelings openly may help to reduce the patient's high level of anxiety.

Mastectomy is no longer the operation of choice for many surgeons, who prefer to remove the lump or sometimes the ovaries, followed by radiotherapy or chemotherapy. With fewer mastectomies being performed you may complete your training without ever caring for a woman who has had to undergo such mutilating surgery. There are many different types of prosthesis that can be slipped into the brassiere which are very effective.

Care plan for patient after removal of breast tissue

Problem	Aim	Nursing care
Potential problem of shock and haemorrhage due to severe fluid loss postoperatively	Prevention or early detection and treatment of shock	Monitor pulse and blood pressure half hourly at first – reduce when stable. Monitor fluid balance carefully. Administer prescribed intravenous fluid/oral input. Monitor tube drainage and report excess. Empty and re-vacuum suction drains when necessary. Check wound for signs of haemorrhage. Check and maintain pressure bandage; repad. Minimize disturbance, move carefully. Sit up when recovered – lean towards affected side to aid drainage.
	Protection and prevention of infection	Leave dressings for 24–48 hours. Aseptic emptying, re-vacuuming and shortening of suction drains. Monitor temperature four hourly – report rise. Observe wound for signs of infection. Ask patient to report pain or excess heat.
Anaesthesia may irritate lungs and potentiate chest infection	Protection from and prevention of chest complications	Encourage deep breathing hourly postoperatively. Involve physiotherapist in expectoration and exercise. Monitor respiratory rate half hourly postoperatively. Observe for signs – haemoptysis, cough. Encourage to sit up. Administer analgesia before chest physiotherapy. Administer steam inhalations four hourly. Assist to expectorate – support wound. Send sputum specimen for culture.
Exacerbation of shock will increase with pain and fear	Prevention of pain and fear exacerbating shock	Explain need for nursing procedures preoperatively to increase understanding and reduce fear. Reassure with known voice that return to ward accomplished safely. Administer prescribed analgesia regularly – four hourly. Adopt most comfortable position – assist to change.
	Minimization of anticipated oedema	Elevate affected arm above level of right atrium. Support with sling or pillows. Check colour and sensation in arm hourly. Take blood pressure, give injections in unaffected arm.
	Prevention of loss of function or deformity	Explain arm will feel stiff at first. Explain plan of gradually increasing movement. Implement plan: First postoperative day – clench and unclench fingers. First 48 hours – full range of movement, i.e. wrist, elbow, arm and shoulder. Encourage to wash face, brush hair and teeth. By 10 days should touch back of neck. Warn to stop if any movement is painful. Report if movement causes pain. **Long-term plan** After skin has healed: Gradually return to household activities. Do not carry heavy items in affected arm. Protect arm from trauma or injury. Do not allow injections or blood pressure measurement to affected arm. Plan rest periods during day and elevate arm. Elevate arm on pillows at night if possible.

Care plan *(continued)*

Problem	Aim	Nursing care
	Patient to work through rejection and anger and come to have positive feelings about altered self-image	Involve partner in discussion of future. Demonstrate prosthesis preoperatively. Involve patient in selection of prosthesis. Invite successful mastectomee to discuss matters. Provide information on clothing – underwear, swimwear. Use soft cotton pad after operation to maintain normal appearance. When wound healed swap for sponge or gel prosthesis. Encourage patient to join in ward activities and not to isolate self. Encourage to look at scar before discharge. Encourage to verbalize feelings. Allow for the release of anger. Understand and accept need to mourn for 'old' self. Provide support and listen to fears.
Fear of rejection due to loss of organ associated with femininity and sexual attraction	Fears openly discussed	Explain no problem concerning hormones, e.g. menopause. Explain about no loss of physical femininity, i.e. stress normal relationships *can* continue. Counsel partner about fears. Encourage discussion of fears and worries. Involve mastectomy nurse if available. Offer psychosexual counselling. Refer to community services for follow-up. Encourage to be up and dressed and return to normality as soon as possible.
Fear of cancer reoccurring/spreading	Early diagnosis and treatment	Explain possibility of future problem and stress need for early detection and reporting of any swelling, redness or pain. Teach to perform breast examination monthly but warn remaining breast tissue will be hard for weeks after operation. Stress importance of out-patient follow-up and continuing treatment, e.g. radiotherapy, when wound has healed.

10.5   Care of the patient with a stoma

For most of us excretion is a very 'personal' matter. Our daily habit, or otherwise, is not something to talk about, and we perform in private behind a locked door even in the home. Patients who are confined to bed and have to use a bedpan find this difficult and embarrassing and often suffer from constipation as a result. In patients with a stoma we have people who have to take even a further step down the ladder of degradation. For not only will they need a nurse to 'empty the bedpan' but to clean up and dress the stoma after the performance which at first they will have no control over. How can society accept them? Even a child can control his bowel movement! As we know, things are not as black as they seem, but we must listen to the patients' fears and apprehensions. Answer their questions honestly and put them in touch with people who have learnt to live successfully with a colostomy. It is good for patients and their partners to talk to others who have been through the experience and learned to live a very full, active and independent life. Careful siting of the stoma on the abdominal wall is essential to ensure the comfortable wearing of the appliance. There are many different appliances on the market and the stoma therapist will help patients choose the best one for their individual needs.

Patients must be given realistic expectations, otherwise they will quickly be discouraged and could become depressed. It is therefore necessary to explain that for the first few days postoperatively the drainage may be fairly free and erratic. Their greatest fear is probably of soiling and odour in public. A sigmoid colostomy may be so well controlled that it resembles normal bowel movement. However, as is the case for all of us, diet, fluid intake and emotional state affects bowel activity and odour.

Diet is affected by taste, custom and culture. Some foods are tolerated better by some than others, but basic high-residue foods are likely to increase bulk and gas content and should therefore be experimented with individually so that the patient can assess their effect. This may include the following foods: onions, celery, sweetcorn, nuts, turnips, prunes, cabbage and pineapple.

Acceptance of the new self-image will come first from the nurse. It is therefore important to keep the patient clean and comfortable without showing any sign of hesitancy or aversion. Self-care will be gradually introduced during which time the patient will need understanding as he reacts and adjusts to his new situation. For details of care for the colostomy patient see Unit 6.

10.6 Care of the patient with altered body image due to other mutilating factors

In a revision book it is not possible to cover all the possible variables of any one theme. In this unit, for example, we have not discussed the care required by a woman following a hysterectomy; a person born with severe skin staining; persons who lose their hair following chemotherapy; severe scarring following radiotherapy, and I am sure you can think of other examples where patients have been distressed as a result of their changed appearance. All these people have one factor in common, they have all suffered a loss, the loss of a perfect body. They will all, to varying degrees, need your support while they grieve (see Unit 11). A few guidelines only can thus be offered to help you care for these patients, but they do not pretend to be complete.

Hysterectomy

Most women need time to adjust following a hysterectomy. If a woman is married and has completed her family the period of grief may be relatively short. However, for a young woman, married or not, the loss of the uterus can be devastating. Gone are her chances of motherhood. Will she still be loved? Will he divorce/leave her? What should they do? In her despair she may turn to many people seeking comfort and solutions. They may contemplate adoption or surrogate motherhood. As a student or pupil nurse you may be the first person to whom they turn, pouring out their feelings. Your main role is to listen and to report to the person in charge who will probably refer the couple to the social worker who is equipped to help them. However, do not fall into the trap of falsely raising the couple's hopes; it does not help in the long run. Remember that the number of healthy, caucasian babies available for adoption is very few. Therefore, the likelihood of the couple being able to adopt such a baby cannot be guaranteed. Surrogate motherhood is not accepted in this country, although there have been reports of people arranging this service for others. It is also very expensive and raises many moral and ethical issues.

Although it may not appear logical (feelings rarely are logical) a single person in her 40s or over may feel the loss of her uterus as intensely as her married counterpart and will need as much support and understanding.

Skin staining

Congenital skin staining, such as the port wine stain, can be very extensive and unsightly. An adult who is admitted to hospital for an unrelated condition has had a lifetime in which to learn to handle his/her reactions to this deformity. However, for many such people entering a new environment it is likely to be difficult for them. On admission they find themselves shut in a ward full of strangers. Over the years they will have developed their own coping mechanisms and they may be very definite in their habits. This can earn them the label of 'a difficult patient'. Sensitive handling on admission, with the nurse taking time to find out the patient's needs, may avoid the trauma that such a label brings both to patients and to nurses (Stockwell, 1972).

Loss of hair

The last body image change that we will mention here is the loss of hair as a result of drugs; this, particularly for women, can be very embarrassing and depressing. The patient may be more concerned about her image than the disease that necessitated the treatment in the first place. The fitting of a wig may help and a sympathetic understanding of the patient's reaction will go a long way.

The one thread that has followed through this unit has been the individual's reaction that has followed a changed body image. This reaction may be very similar to that following bereavement which is studied in the next unit.

For a quick and easy revision test on this unit see page 117.

References

Stockwell, F., *The Unpopular Patient* (RCN, 1972)

Further reading

Delvin, D., *A Patient's Guide to Operations* (Penguin, 1981)

Muir, I. F. and Barclay, T. L., *Burns and their Treatment* (Lloyd-Luke, 1974)

Robinson, N. and Swash, I., *Mastectomy: A Patient's Guide to Coping with Breast Surgery* (Thorsons, 1977)

Fisher, S. H., *Psychiatric Considerations of Hand Disability* (*Archives of Physical Medicine and Rehabilitation*, **41**, 1960)

11 Care of the dying patient and relatives

11.1 Introduction

The customs surrounding death and dying are culturally orientated. In the western world we seem to deny death. It has become a taboo subject, and doctors may feel they have failed if the patient dies. Evelyn Waugh (1977) has portrayed the western attitude to death in his book *The Loved One*.

However, the definition of nursing quoted in Unit 1 states that one of the duties of the nurse is to help the patient to a peaceful death. How can we do this if we deny its occurrence? It is very difficult for a young nurse to know what to say and how to care for dying patients and their relatives because of their lack of experience. They may never have experienced bereavement or been closely involved with a family that has.

11.2 Grief

People like Parkes (1975) and Kübler-Ross (1970) have made a study of the subject of grief and loss and conclude that the experience need not be ultimately destructive but can bring strength and maturity. Parkes (1975) identifies seven major features that may be observed in many bereavement reactions. These are:

1 A process of realization – denial – avoidance towards acceptance;
2 Alarm reaction – anxiety, restlessness, fear;
3 Urge to search and find lost person;
4 Anger and guilt;
5 Feelings of internal loss of self or mutilation;
6 Identification phenomena with dead person, such as feeling him or her close at hand;
7 Pathological variants.

Fisher (1960) and others suggest that people suffering mutilation (altered body image – see Unit 10) pass through a similar process of mourning.

Kübler-Ross describes five stages of grief. It is helpful for us to know these stages as it will help us in our understanding. Although five stages are described there may be some overlap of the stages; that is patients will not necessarily complete stage 1 before passing to stage 2. For grief to be a healing process it is necessary to pass through all five stages. For people who stick at one of the earlier stages, grief becomes destructive and counselling is required to help reduce the damage caused.

The five stages of grief according to Kübler-Ross are:

1 Denial
2 Anger
3 Bargaining
4 Depression
5 Acceptance

The family and the patient go through similar stages of grieving but they are not necessarily at the same stage at the same time, which creates difficulties. These five stages have been used by the hospice movement to train their counsellors and at St. Christopher's, Sydenham, London, they have reduced the stages to four in the following way:

1 Numbness or denial that death has occurred
2 Searching, often accompanied by strong feelings of anger and guilt
3 Disorganization and despair
4 Reorganization and establishment of purpose in the life that is left

What has this to do with caring for the dying patient? There is a process that is called 'anticipatory grief'. People who know they are dying need to grieve for the life that they will lose, for the work that is yet unaccomplished, to see the children off their hands, etc, as much as relatives need to grieve for the one who dies. Both parties will need to pass through the four stages of grief described. By enabling our patient to come to terms with his or her own death we will be helping him or her to come to the 'peaceful death' described by Henderson.

Before we can help others come to terms with human frailty in the form of death, we need to examine our own anxieties, fears and attitudes to death. If we do not do this, our feelings are likely to get in the way and make caring for the dying and their relatives difficult for us. Some hospitals run terminal care support teams, and part of their work is to support the nurses caring for dying patients. To help you sort out your own feelings, preferably before you are confronted with the situation on the ward, try to join a small discussion group led by specialists such as a sister from the terminal care team, a nurse counsellor or the chaplain. Death is a part of life, and the more you are able to talk about it, openly discussing your feelings, the easier you will find it to talk and discuss the subject with your patients.

Just as you need to talk about the subject, so do your patients, but perhaps in a different way. When the truth of the diagnosis or prognosis has sunk in, the patient is likely to become very angry, asking – 'why me?'. The question may be asked many times in many different ways. They may lash out at the medical and nursing staff – 'why can't you cure me?'. They may go in search of a cure if their condition permits. Perhaps they will seek a second medical opinion, or a visit to a herbalist or a 'healer'. This search for a cure may be accompanied by feelings of guilt – 'if only I hadn't . . .'. There is no answer as such, but the expression of their feeling of guilt may help. If acceptable, a minister of religion can be consulted. When alternative means of cure also fail and their general condition is obviously deteriorating they may become depressed, full of despair and not know what to do next. With help, support and quiet understanding the patient will hopefully come to acceptance and make the best of what life is left to them.

No time scale can be placed on these four stages; some patients will die while still angry, while others may come through to acceptance relatively quickly. The patient's attitude to death will affect the time scale, for instance those with a strong religious faith may come to acceptance more quickly than others. The patient and relatives, however, must be allowed to grieve. By this I mean to be emotionally involved, to be in touch with their feelings and be free to express them. Unfortunately, in our culture, showing emotion is frowned upon. Patients, relatives and staff need to be given privacy and space to encourage them to express their feelings. Acceptance by the staff of tears – even from men – is essential. They are not a sign of weakness, but the beginning of healing.

11.3   Bereavement

Bereavement is a crisis point in one's life, causing exceptional stress. The bereaved person will go over and over the circumstances surrounding the death. They need to be able to do this, as it is part of the healing process. Therefore if you can lend an ear, even if you have heard the story before, you will be helping the bereaved relative. You do not usually need to say anything, just listen, and show you are listening. Try not to send the relative home to an empty house. Contact other members of the family. The support of a caring family or friends who can share the grief will help to heal the wound. They will also need to care physically for the bereaved person who may be reluctant to prepare meals and to eat.

Where there is no family or friends the remaining relative is particularly at risk. A bereavement counsellor or visitor should be contacted as quickly as possible. Where it is known that when the patient dies the relative will be alone, the bereavement counsellor or visitor should be contacted so that they can establish a relationship before the death occurs.

Caring for the dying is very demanding but rewarding work. There are now courses available to teach nurses how to care for the dying. These are available as post-registration courses and are usually run by specialist hostels or hospices, such as St. Joseph's, Hackney, and St. Christopher's, Sydenham, in London and Dorothy House Foundation, Bath.

Care plan for a dying patient

Problem	Aim	Nursing care
Increasing inability to perform physical care activities	Provision of physical care with regard to patients' needs and ability in accordance with their own wishes	Consult patient and elicit wishes. Involve patient in care planning. Respect wishes wherever possible. Explain to patient reasons for planned action. Allow the patient to do as much as he wishes for him/herself.

Care plan (*continued*)

Problem	Aim	Nursing
Fear of loss of independence and self-esteem	Prevention of distressing complications	Provide remainder of care in the following areas: skin; eyes; mouth; hair; pressure areas; diet and fluids; elimination; nausea and vomiting. Check on patient's satisfaction with care. (See care plans in Unit 9.)
Fear of isolation and dying alone	Provision of security and companionship Giving some time for quiet thinking	Wherever possible, one nurse or team should care for patient. Develop relationship of trust – answer questions honestly. Be available if needed. Give prompt attention if summoned – do not avoid patient. Ensure frequent physical presence, not just when actual care given. Provide contact – hold hand. Provide some hope of relief.
Fear of pain and suffering (see Unit 8, care plan)	Relief from pain, if possible without clouding consciousness Identification of other problems which may increase pain:	Check pain not anxiety related. Explore with patient best method of pain relief. Involve patient in decision making. Administer medication before pain perceived. Increase dosage/change medication if indicated. Record reaction to analgesia. Check for other physical discomfort and relieve if possible
	Ensure sleep and rest	Bed in quiet position in ward. Provide quiet periods to rest. Use night sedation if indicated.
	Emotional worries	Provide calm relaxed atmosphere and open communication so fears can be expressed and discussed.
Fear of the unknown	Alleviation of anxiety and provision of support	Encourage discussion of beliefs. Involve spiritual adviser if helpful. Discuss ideas of death. Encourage expression of fears. Avoid false reassurances.
Coping with death	Patient moves through stages at own pace, from: denial/shock; anger; bargaining; depression; acceptance; to peaceful death	Check patient awareness of prognosis and likely course of events. Liaise between patient, family and physician to check knowledge and understanding of situation. Assess which stage patient is at and provide necessary care. Encourage frank and open discussion. Provide calm, relaxed, caring atmosphere so patient can express ideas and work through process. Do not attempt to hurry on to next stage. Provide emotional support.
Coping with the family	Family will cope with prognosis and be supportive to dying patient – anticipate their needs to prevent distress	Assess understanding and knowledge – provide information. Be available for discussion and support. Observe for evidence of inability to cope – explore their beliefs, expectations and attitudes to death; check for feelings of guilt. Prepare family for stages of dying and bereavement. Work with them through grieving process and support them by counselling. Provide privacy for relatives to express their grief. Allow to participate in care if desired. Keep them informed in their absence. After the death allow them to express grief and mourn.

For a quick and easy revision test on this unit turn to page 118.

References

Bayly, J., *The Last Thing We Talk About* (Cook, 1973)
Fisher, S. H., *Psychiatric Considerations of Hand Disability* (Archives of Physical Medicine and Rehabilitation, 1960)
Kübler-Ross, E., *On Death and Dying* (Tavistock, 1970)
Parkes, C. M., *Bereavement: studies of grief in adult life* (Penguin, 1975)
Waugh, E., *The Loved One* (Little, 1977)

Further reading

Kübler-Ross, E., *The Final Stage of Growth* (Prentice Hall, 1975)
Kübler-Ross, E., *To Live Until We Say Goodbye* (Prentice Hall, 1978)
Kübler-Ross, E., *Living with Death and Dying* (Souvenir Press, 1982)
Lewis, C. S., *A Grief Observed* (Faber and Faber, 1966)
Vanauken, S., *A Severe Mercy* (Harper Row, 1980)

Section III

Self-test units

Unit 1

1 Which one of the following **best** describes the term 'health':
   (a) absence of disease or infirmity
   (b) ability to perform activities of living independently
   (c) the correct response to life's stress
   (d) being neither well nor ill

2 Which of the following **best** describes the term 'health education':
   (a) instruction of the public how to use the Health Service
   (b) monitoring the nation's health state
   (c) prevention of sickness occurring
   (d) pre-symptomatic detection of diseases

3 Which of the following is the process by which effective communication occurs? A message is:
   (a) perceived, conveyed, received and understood
   (b) conveyed, received, perceived and interpreted
   (c) received, decoded, understood and perceived
   (d) encoded, understood, recoded and received

4 Which of the following is the usual sequence of the stages of the nursing process:
   (a) history taking, planning, problem identification, assessment
   (b) assessment, implementation, history taking, evaluation
   (c) problem identification, planning, assessment, documentation
   (d) assessment, planning, implementation, evaluation

5 Which one of the following skills would be **most** useful to the nurse in the assessment stage of the nursing process:
   (a) interpersonal communication
   (b) clinical expertise   (c) logical reasoning   (d) problem solving

6 Which of the following is recognized as the main aim of the nursing process? To:
   (a) ensure good nurse-to-nurse communication
   (b) improve nursing record keeping
   (c) meet an individual's need for care
   (d) make nurses accountable for their actions

7 Which of the following, according to Henderson's (1966) definition, is nursing:
   (a) the major caring profession
   (b) a service for the sick and dying
   (c) providing care for the dependent and needy
   (d) helping people in need to health, recovery or a peaceful death

8 Which of the following would be considered 'safety needs' according to Maslow's (1954) theory? The need for:
   (a) fulfilment of potential, human development
   (b) recognition of worth and dignity
   (c) freedom from fear, structure and stability
   (d) love and respect from others

9 Which one of the following actions should a nurse take if a patient refuses to co-operate with care which has been planned:
   (a) tell the patient the care planner is experienced and knows best
   (b) explain fully the reason why the action is needed
   (c) report the incident to the senior nurse on duty
   (d) record on the plan that the patient refused care

10 Which of the following best explains independence? A state where:
   (a) a person copes with daily living unaided
   (b) other people are involved in organizing daily living
   (c) some functions are dealt with by care givers
   (d) an individual lives within his own limits

Unit 2

1 Which of the following statements is true:
 (a) digestion of nutrients is completed by the stomach
 (b) nutrients are absorbed mainly in the colon
 (c) the gall bladder secretes the digestive enzyme bile
 (d) peristaltic movement propels food by muscular contraction

2 Which of the following structures is the appendix attached to:
 (a) ileum
 (b) caecum
 (c) colon
 (d) jejunum

3 Which of the following statements is true:
 (a) the appetite centre is the medulla in the brain stem
 (b) the basic metabolic rate is controlled by the hypothalamus
 (c) glucocorticoids increase the breakdown of protein
 (d) weight gain is due to excessive protein intake

4 Which of the following dietary regimens is the *most* appropriate for a pyrexial patient:
 (a) increased calories and fluids, reduced fat
 (b) decreased calories and vitamins, increased minerals
 (c) increased vitamins and minerals, reduced fat
 (d) increased protein and fluids, increased minerals

5 Which of the following describes the principles of total parenteral nutrition? Provision of nutrients via a(n):
 (a) enterostomy tube
 (b) fine bore nasogastric tube
 (c) fibreoptic scope
 (d) intravenous catheter

6 Which of the following is the reason glucocorticoids are prescribed for patients suffering from ulcerative colitis? In order to:
 (a) reduce inflammation
 (b) raise blood glucose levels
 (c) increase potassium excretion
 (d) improve peristalsis

7 Which of the following pieces of advice should the nurse give to patients before a barium meal? They/their:
 (a) stools may be pale and float in the pan afterwards
 (b) will be starved for 12 hours afterwards
 (c) should expect loose stools for 24 hours
 (d) pulse and blood pressure will be monitored four hourly

8 Which of the following describes malabsorption due to coeliac disease:
 (a) difficulty in digesting cellulose
 (b) increased speed of nutrients through the intestines
 (c) inability to obtain nutrients due to damaged mucosa
 (d) absence of essential digestive enzymes

9 Which one of the following is the main reason for obesity in the western world? A(n):
 (a) inadequate carbohydrate metabolism
 (b) excessive consumption of calories
 (c) underactive thyroid gland
 (d) failure in the production of amino acids

10 Which one of the following menus would be **most** suitable for a patient prescribed a 1000 calorie a day diet:
 (a) 8 oz grilled lean steak, green salad and boiled potatoes
 (b) chicken and vegetable casserole and 4 oz fried rice
 (c) 6 oz white fish in cheese sauce, peas with two slices brown bread
 (d) two poached eggs, two rashers of grilled bacon, tomatoes and mushrooms

Unit 3

1 Which of the following observations would lead a nurse to suspect a patient is dehydrated:
 (a) hypertension, bradycardia, polyuria, weight loss

    (b) wrinkled skin, hypotension, tachycardia, polyuria

    (c) oliguria, wrinkled skin, hypertension, bradycardia

    (d) weight loss, tachycardia, oliguria, hypotension.

2 Which one of the following actions should the nurse take if a patient receiving an intravenous infusion complains of breathlessness, headache and palpitations:

    (a) monitor the respiratory rate half hourly

    (b) change the infusion solution

    (c) stop the infusion

    (d) weigh the patient daily

3 Which of the following statements is true:

    (a) blood filters through the glomerulus into the Bowman's capsules

    (b) the loop of Henle dips down into the renal cortex

    (c) cells in the convoluted tubule reabsorb water

    (d) aldosterone controls urea secretion

4 Which of the following describes the process of urine formation:

    (a) diffusion, reabsorption, excretion

    (b) filtration, selective reabsorption, secretion

    (c) filtration, assimilation, collection

    (d) collection, selective absorption, filtration

5 Which one of the following terms describes the process by which water molecules move from an area of low concentration to a high concentration solution through a semi-permeable membrane:

    (a) osmosis

    (b) diffusion

    (c) homeostasis

    (d) absorption

6 Which of the following events would occur if a patient was losing or not producing plasma proteins:

    (a) increased tissue fluid formation

    (b) arterial blood pressure would rise steeply

    (c) less lymph would be produced

    (d) venous pressure would increase

7 Which of the following urinary outputs should the nurse report immediately:

    (a) 60 ml per hour

    (b) 0.06 litres per hour

    (c) 300 ml in 24 hours

    (d) 1.5 litres in 24 hours

8 Which of the following observations would provide the **best** information about a patient's fluid balance:

    (a) four hourly urinalysis

    (b) daily weight

    (c) eight hourly urinalysis

    (d) daily urine output

9 Which of the following would be **most** useful advice to a patient suffering from diarrhoea:

    (a) restrict the intake of salt in the diet

    (b) increase their intake of strong black coffee

    (c) reduce the amount of glucose-containing food

    (d) drink plenty of Bovril and fruit juice

Unit 4

1 Which of the following blood vessels transports blood from the right ventricle to the lungs:

    (a) intercostal artery

    (b) pulmonary artery

    (c) pulmonary vein

    (d) intercostal vein

2 Which of the following structures consists of a wall of single cells:

    (a) alveolus

    (b) areolar

    (c) bronchiole

    (d) lobule

3 Which of the following is the primary stimulant for the respiratory centre:
   (a) phrenic nerve impulses
   (b) cerebral cortex
   (c) oxygen
   (d) carbon dioxide
4 Which of the following occurs during the process of respiration:
   (a) oxygen and carbon dioxide diffuse from areas of high to areas of low concentration
   (b) oxygen and carbon dioxide diffuse from areas of low to areas of high concentration
   (c) carbon dioxide molecules combine with haemoglobin
   (d) oxyhaemoglobin releases. oxygen molecules
5 Which of the following describes the difference between inspired and expired air? Inspired air contains:
   (a) equal percentages of carbon dioxide and nitrogen
   (b) more carbon dioxide and less oxygen
   (c) increased percentages of oxygen and carbon dioxide
   (d) more oxygen and less carbon dioxide
6 Which of the following terms should a nurse use to describe a patient experiencing difficulty breathing in and out:
   (a) orthopnoea
   (b) cyanosis
   (c) dyspnoea
   (d) stridor
7 Which of the following plans of care would be most helpful to a patient suffering breathlessness due to congestive cardiac failure? An oxygen concentration that is:
   (a) high and rest flat in bed
   (b) low and increase active movements
   (c) high and improve blood circulation
   (d) low and sit upright
8 Which of the following is the reason that patients suffering from bronchitis are prescribed low oxygen percentages? It:
   (a) prevents over-breathing of oxygen
   (b) reduces the lungs' vital capacity
   (c) improves normal oxygen pressure in the lungs
   (d) maintains the stimulus to the respiratory centre
9 Which of the following is the reason smoking is prohibited in an area where oxygen is being administered:
   (a) oxygen supports combustion
   (b) sparks may set bedding alight
   (c) other patients may object
   (d) smoke pollutes the atmosphere
10 Which of the following actions should the nurse take if the patient she is giving a steam inhalation to is frail and unsteady:
   (a) ensure the inhaler is properly assembled
   (b) stay with the patient throughout the procedure
   (c) make the inhalation temperature much lower
   (d) place the air inlet away from the patient

Unit 5

1 Which of the following is correct:
   (a) renin is produced in the vasomotor centre
   (b) angiotensin increases sodium and water reabsorption
   (c) during stress adrenaline is secreted by the adrenal cortex
   (d) peripheral resistance occurs mainly in the venules
2 Which of the following is correct? Blood pressure falls if:
   (a) control of the vasomotor centre is lost
   (b) blood becomes more viscous
   (c) peripheral resistance is high
   (d) cardiac output is increased

3 Which of the following observations would indicate that a patient was in a state of shock? Pulse rate:
   (a) slow and weak, colour flushed, and drowsy
   (b) rapid and weak, colour pale, and clammy
   (c) slow and strong, colour pale, and listless
   (d) rapid and strong, colour flushed, and restless

4 Which of the following describes myocardial infarction:
   (a) intense pain in the chest on inspiration, not relieved by rest
   (b) interruption of blood supply to cardiac muscle
   (c) irregular heart rhythm due to low blood pressure
   (d) due to massive vasodilation of the coronary artery

5 Which of the following describes the priorities of resuscitation of a collapsed patient:
   (a) circulation, breathing, airway
   (b) airway, circulation, breathing
   (c) breathing, airway, circulation
   (d) airway, breathing, circulation

6 Which of the following is the main principle of management of a patient with haematemesis:
   (a) keep warm with extra blankets
   (b) encourage oral fluids to replace lost fluid
   (c) apply pressure and elevate the part
   (d) elevate head on one pillow and keep calm

7 Which one of the following observations would indicate a patient is reacting adversely to a blood transfusion:
   (a) skin rash, fevered brow, tingling in fingertips, dyspnoea
   (b) pallor, shivering, tingling in fingers, dyspnoea
   (c) skin rash, headache, chest and back pain, dyspnoea
   (d) erythema, fevered brow, chest and back pain, tachypnoea

8 Which of the following events occurs when blood clots:
   (a) lymphocytes plug the damaged vessel
   (b) prothrombin is released from damaged cells
   (c) fibrinogen breaks down to form fibrin
   (d) blood cells become tangled in the meshwork of fibres

9 Which of the following actions should the nurse take if when admitting a patient his diastolic pressure is 110 mm Hg.
   (a) record his blood pressure lying and standing every 4 hours
   (b) order a low-fat diet and advise weight loss
   (c) ask patient to rest and repeat the recording in half hour
   (d) order complete bed rest and elevate the foot of the bed

Unit 6

1 Which of the following is the main function of the colon:
   (a) secretion of vitamins B and K
   (b) breakdown of amino acids
   (c) absorption of water
   (d) formation of gases

2 Which of the following describes the normal process of defaecation in the adult:
   (a) under control of the parasympathetic nervous system
   (b) a spinal reflex which the higher centres have gained control of
   (c) under control of the sympathetic nervous system
   (d) a reflex action controlled by the sacral nerve plexus

3 Which of the following statements is correct:
   (a) diarrhoea occurs due to loss of control of the internal sphincter
   (b) decreased peristalsis is associated with irritable bowel syndrome
   (c) straining at stool is due to inadequate metabolism of cellulose
   (d) repeated failure to relax the external sphincter leads to constipation

4 Which of the following describes the action of glycerine suppositories:
   (a) bulk additive
   (b) contact purgative
   (c) faecal softener
   (d) osmotic diuretic

5 Which of the following is true? A colostomy in the descending colon:
   (a) will function throughout the night and day
   (b) will inevitably produce odour from the bag
   (c) should have a 3 cm space around the stoma
   (d) should be cleaned with soap and water

6 Which of the following statements is true:
   (a) normal micturition in the adult is achieved by spinal reflex
   (b) incontinence occurs due to loss of sphincter control
   (c) enuresis occurs because the bladder trigone is inadequate
   (d) catheterization will improve incontinence

7 Which of the following observations should the nurse report **immediately** on a patient 24 hours after prostatectomy:
   (a) haematuria
   (b) catheter appears to be leaking
   (c) cloudy urine
   (d) catheter drainage ceasing

8 Which of the following is the correct method for catheter hygiene:
   (a) scrub up and down firmly to remove all encrustation
   (b) use cotton-wool balls for each swabbing to and from the urethra
   (c) wipe away from the urethral outlet with soap and water
   (d) use alcohol-impregnated wipes and gloves around the urethra

9 Which of the following plans would be **most** useful if a nurse suspects that a patient with a catheter has a urinary infection:
   (a) increase fluid input and send a specimen of urine to laboratory
   (b) change catheter aseptically and perform catheter hygiene four hourly
   (c) send a specimen of urine to laboratory then administer antibiotics
   (d) perform bladder wash-out and catheter hygiene four hourly

Unit 7

1 Which of the following statements is correct? A body temperature of:
   (a) 35.5 °C is termed hypothermia
   (b) 36.8 °C is considered normal for an adult
   (c) 37 °C is termed a pyrexia
   (d) 42 °C is compatible with cell functioning

2 Which one of the following processes increases the amount ot heat loss from the body:
   (a) condensation
   (b) conservation
   (c) convection
   (d) constriction

3 Which one of the following is the main source of body heat:
   (a) chemical breakdown of foodstuffs
   (b) shivering
   (c) heat-regulating centre
   (d) environment

4 Which of the following statements is correct? Body temperature is:
   (a) lower in the axilla than the mouth
   (b) higher in the groin than the axilla
   (c) lowest in the rectum
   (d) higher in the morning than the evening

5 Which of the following is the correct principle in caring for a hypothermic patient:
   (a) correct any dehydration urgently
   (b) keep the room temperature at a constant 36 °C
   (c) rewarm as rapidly as possible
   (d) increase the core temperature by 0.5°C hourly

6 Which one of the following substances initiates phagocytosis when it is released from injured cells:
   (a) fibrinogen
   (b) antigen
   (c) histamine
   (d) neutrophil

7 Which of the following are the cardinal signs of inflammation:
   (a) pus, pain, pallor, oedema, decreased blood supply
   (b) heat, pus, pain, swelling, loss of sensation
   (c) pain, oedema, pus, pallor, decreased nerve supply
   (d) heat, redness, pain, swelling, loss of function

8 Which of the following is the **best** way a nurse can prevent cross-infection:
   (a) isolating infected patients
   (b) routinely culturing open wounds
   (c) handwashing before and after patient contact
   (d) teaching patients about hygiene and health

9 Which one of the following is the reason patients suffering tuberculosis are barrier nursed? To prevent spread of infection by:
   (a) direct contact
   (b) airborne transmission
   (c) a fomite
   (d) a vehicle

10 Which of the following is the reason patients suffering leukaemia are nursed in protective isolation? Because/to:
   (a) the white cell count is raised
   (b) prevent the transmission of infection via fomites
   (c) their immune system cannot react to microbial invasion
   (d) increase their resistance to micro-organisms

Unit 8

1 Which of the following is the best description of pain:
   (a) the sensation a patient perceives
   (b) a specific nervous stimulus
   (c) a sensory input of known quantity
   (d) impulses originating from the tactile corpuscles

2 Which one of the following statements about pain is correct? Pain:
   (a) is non-functional and undesirable
   (b) varies according to mood, experience and culture
   (c) is related to the amount of tissue damage
   (d) can be located precisely to an area

3 Which one of the following describes the body's immediate reaction to a painful stimulus, for example, touching a naked flame:
   (a) sensory impulse
   (b) withdrawal reflex
   (c) spinothalamic arc
   (d) perceptive withdrawal

4 Which of the following explains the gate control theory of pain? Sensory input is:
   (a) regulated by the spinothalamic tract
   (a) free to enter the sensory cortex
   (c) blocked at the dorsal horn cells
   (d) transmitted to the motor cortex if impulses strong enough

5 Which of the following is the morphine-like substance produced by the body as its own pain reliever:
   (a) endorphin

(b) cyclomorphine
(c) endoplasm
(d) bradykinin

6 Which of the following describes referred pain? Pain that:
(a) is limited to a specific body area
(b) is impossible to pinpoint
(c) is perceived as coming from the deeper tissues
(d) results from stimulation of superficial fibres

7 Which of the following is the best way to treat a patient suffering chronic pain:
(a) reassure them that things will improve
(b) offer pain relief when necessary
(c) try to distract their attention
(d) administer prescribed analgesia at regular intervals

8 Which of the following factors is most likely to lower a patient's pain threshold:
(a) sympathy and understanding
(b) diversions
(c) fear and anxiety
(d) relaxation

9 Which one of the following reactions cannot be voluntarily controlled in a patient suffering pain:
(a) weeping
(b) grinding teeth
(c) facial grimacing
(d) perspiring

10 Which of the following is the effect morphine has on pain:
(a) inhibits pain perception in the dorsal horn cell
(b) slows the impulse up the spinothalamic tracts
(c) depresses the local perception of sensation
(d) enhances the body's production of natural pain relievers

Unit 9

1 Which of the following covers the articulating surfaces of a bone at a synovial joint:
(a) capsular ligament
(b) hyaline cartilage
(c) ciliated epithelium
(d) synovial membrane

2 Which of the following structures joins a muscle to a bone:
(a) cartilage
(b) ligament
(c) membrane
(d) tendon

3 Which of the following statements about osteoarthritis is true? It:
(a) is a non-inflammatory degenerative joint condition
(b) commonly affects women in their 40s
(c) is a chronic inflammatory disorder of weight-bearing joints
(d) is a painless swelling of the capsular ligaments

4 Which of the following are patients suffering rheumatoid arthritis likely to demonstrate:
(a) no improvement after steroid treatment
(b) pain in the weight-bearing joints
(c) swollen joints and general malaise
(d) increased joint mobility and function

5 Which of the following is the function of traction in a fracture of the lower limb? In order to:
(a) prevent weight bearing
(b) elevate the limb
(c) exert pressure and prevent displacement
(d) oppose the body weight by counterbalance

6 Which of the following is correct? Weights may be removed from the traction apparatus if:
   (a) the patient needs to go for X-ray
   (b) passing urine uphill becomes a problem
   (c) during bed making the weight may swing
   (d) the patient experiences severe pain

7 Which one of the following is the nurse's priority when dealing with a newly paralysed patient:
   (a) vocational and diversional therapy
   (b) improving and retraining unaffected muscles
   (c) overcoming the stress of the condition
   (d) establishing a new daily routine

8 Which of the following plans would be **most** useful to a patient suffering right-sided hemiplegia:
   (a) full range of passive exercises two or three times daily
   (b) active exercise of all limbs three times daily
   (c) muscle strengthening exercises for the right limbs
   (d) bilateral straight leg raising exercises

9 Which of the following plans would most help a patient with aphasia:
   (a) speak slowly and loudly
   (b) use gestures to reinforce meanings
   (c) accept what the patient says is correct
   (d) encourage him to write down what he wants

10 Which of the following plans would assist in the rehabilitation of a patient after a cerebral vascular accident:
   (a) keep working on skills until they are perfected
   (b) accept that independent existence is impossible
   (c) total nursing care for the first week
   (d) encourage any attempts to assist in care activities

Unit 10

1 Which one of the following is the best description of 'body image':
   (a) the way other people perceive us
   (b) an ideal figure to aim for
   (c) what we see reflected in the mirror
   (d) the picture we have of ourselves

2 Which one of the following is the best way for a nurse to react to a physical disfigurement in a patient she is admitting:
   (a) obtain full details by direct questioning
   (b) ignore the disfigurement and carry on as usual
   (c) allow the subject to emerge naturally if possible
   (d) plan to make enquires from a relative

3 Which of the following is true:
   (a) bacteriocides will remove pathogens from the dermis
   (b) intact skin prevents invasion by micro-organisms
   (c) granules of the pigment melanin protect against ultraviolet radiation
   (d) sebaceous glands aid in the excretion of waste products

4 Which of the following is the nurse's priority when caring for a patient suffering second-degree burns:
   (a) monitor blood pressure and pulse hourly to assess shock
   (b) prevent heat loss and reduce body temperature
   (c) order a high protein and vitamin diet and push fluids
   (d) passive movements to prevent contractures and scarring

5 Which of the following is the reason why patients who have undergone a mid-thigh amputation are encouraged to lie prone for half an hour four times daily? To:
   (a) ensure optimum stump shape
   (b) improve circulation in remaining tissue
   (c) reduce stump oedema and swelling
   (d) prevent flexion contractures occurring

6 Which of the following is the best way the nurse can help a patient experiencing phantom pain after the amputation:
   (a) divert the focus of attention to the other limbs
   (b) check daily the stump has not become oedematous
   (c) administer analgesia until the sensation ceases
   (d) explain why pain cannot occur if a limb is absent

7 Which of the following is a common complication following a mastectomy:
   (a) gynaecomastia
   (b) lymphoedema
   (c) mastitis
   (d) papilloedema

8 Which of the following should the nurse advise a patient after a mastectomy before discharge home:
   (a) not to wear the prosthesis when swimming
   (b) to offer the affected arm for blood pressure recordings
   (c) not to carry heavy things with the affected arm
   (d) to get back to full arm mobility as soon as possible

9 Which of the following actions should the nurse take when dealing with a patient with a newly formed colostomy who appears revulsed by their stoma:
   (a) enlist their help with small tasks associated with stoma care
   (b) explain that no one else will notice or need know
   (c) show them exactly what it looks like in a mirror
   (d) avoid discussing the stoma while dealing with it

10 Which of the following should the nurse advise a patient with a newly formed permanent colostomy before discharge home:
   (a) to avoid swimming and going out to dinner frequently
   (b) eat plenty of fruit and continue playing football carefully
   (c) change to a sedentary job and eat a high-residue diet
   (d) to identify their own food tolerance and take moderate exercise

Unit 11

1 Which one of the following describes the principles of care for patients who are dying:
   (a) maintenance of appearance and dignity
   (b) promotion of physical and mental comfort
   (c) prevention of complications of immobility
   (d) alleviation of fear and anxiety

2 Which of the following, according to Kübler-Ross, are the stages of dying:
   (a) denial, anger, bargaining, despair, acceptance
   (b) anger, guilt, despair, bargaining, denial
   (c) denial, guilt, despair, grief, enlightenment
   (d) anger, despondence, denial, despair, acceptance

3 Which of the following best describes grief:
   (a) depression following an unpleasant experience
   (b) negative attitude to death or loss
   (c) part of the healing process after loss
   (d) a feeling of guilt for things left undone

4 Which of the following actions should the nurse take if another member of staff appears to be upset by a patient's death:
   (a) wait until later to broach the subject
   (b) ask whether she would like to discuss it
   (c) ignore the subject until the nurse mentions it
   (d) keep a professional distance from her

5 Which of the following aims should be the nurse's priority when caring for a patient who is dying:
   (a) strict two-hourly turns to prevent pressure sores
   (b) promotion of maximum independence
   (c) high-fibre diet to avoid constipation
   (d) allow patient to participate in care planning

6 Which of the following is the reason for hospice care? To:
   (a) prevent dying patients upsetting others
   (b) allow relatives open visiting
   (c) ensure an individual's needs are fulfilled
   (d) provide a peaceful environment

7 Which of the following actions should the nurse take if a patient with carcinoma asks her if he is going to die:
   (a) remind him that everyone has to die eventually
   (b) ask the minister to talk to the patient
   (c) tell him to ask the doctors next time they call
   (d) check the situation with a senior nurse and return to the patient

8 Which of the following actions should the nurse take if a patient who is terminally ill reports feeling hopeless and sees no point in living:
   (a) sit down and listen to his reasons for this statement
   (b) tell him to stop talking like that and pull himself together
   (c) reassure him that things are never as bad as they seem
   (d) make him a cup of tea and try and cheer him up

9 Which of the following would be **most** useful in supporting a dying patient's relatives:
   (a) ensure that they are not alone at home frequently
   (b) keep them informed and telephone them if his condition changes
   (c) offer cups of tea and a quiet place to sit after visiting
   (d) be available and willing to discuss their feelings

10 Which of the following is the correct procedure following a patient's death:
   (a) inform the nursing officer, remove dentures and jewellery, prop up the chin, cover with a sheet
   (b) notify the mortician, pack all orifices, support the jaw, leave half an hour
   (c) call the doctor, remove dentures, make up a clean bed, move the body to mortuary
   (d) note the time, close the eyes, lay the patient flat, return in 1 hour

Answers to self-test units

Unit 1

1(b) 2(c) 3(b) 4(d) 5(a) 6(c) 7(d) 8(c) 9(b) 10(a)

Unit 2

1(d) 2(b) 3(c) 4(a) 5(d) 6(a) 7(a) 8(d) 9(b) 10(a)

Unit 3

1(d) 2(c) 3(c) 4(b) 5(a) 6(a) 7(c) 8(b) 9(d)

Unit 4

1(b) 2(a) 3(d) 4(a) 5(d) 6(c) 7(d) 8(d) 9(a) 10(b)

Unit 5

1(b) 2(a) 3(b) 4(b) 5(d) 6(d) 7(c) 8(d) 9(c)

Unit 6

1(c) 2(b) 3(d) 4(c) 5(d) 6(c) 7(d) 8(c) 9(a)

Unit 7

1(b) 2(c) 3(a) 4(a) 5(d) 6(c) 7(d) 8(c) 9(b) 10(c)

Unit 8

1(a) 2(b) 3(b) 4(c) 5(a) 6(b) 7(d) 8(c) 9(d) 10(a)

Unit 9

1(b) 2(d) 3(a) 4(c) 5(c) 6(d) 7(c) 8(a) 9(b) 10(d)

Unit 10

1(d) 2(c) 3(b) 4(a) 5(d) 6(c) 7(b) 8(c) 9(a) 10(d)

Unit 11

1(b) 2(a) 3(c) 4(b) 5(d) 6(c) 7(d) 8(a) 9(d) 10(d)

Section IV

Practice tests

Practice test 1

1 Which one of the following actions should the nurse take if, when admitting a patient, she discovers a diastolic blood pressure of 110 mm Hg:
   (a) ask the doctor to check the reading
   (b) repeat the recording with the patient lying down
   (c) tell the patient his blood pressure is high
   (d) check the recording after the patient has settled in

2 Which of the following is recognized as the main aim of the nursing process? To:
   (a) ensure tasks are not forgotten
   (b) improve nurse teaching
   (c) provide care according to need
   (d) supply a format for record keeping

3 Which of the following is the best way a nurse can prevent cross-infection? By:
   (a) enforcing strict isolation nursing procedures
   (b) preceding patient contact with handwashing
   (c) performing aseptic techniques correctly
   (d) keeping hair tidy and nails short

4 Which one of the following is the primary stimulant for the respiratory centre:
   (a) impulses from the phrenic nerve
   (b) carbon dioxide levels
   (c) impulses to the cerebral cortex
   (d) oxygen levels

5 Which one of the following unites bone and muscle:
   (a) tendon
   (b) white fibrous tissue
   (c) yellow elastic fibres
   (d) cartilage

6 Which one of the following is the first-aider's priority when caring for a patient who has first-degree burns of the palm:
   (a) apply a cooling lanolin-based cream
   (b) cover with a non-adhesive dressing
   (c) place an ice-pack onto the area
   (d) immerse the hand in cool water

7 Which of the following is the nurse's priority when caring for an elderly lady with myxoedema who is admitted in a collapsed state with a temperature of 35 °C:
   (a) increase core temperature by 0.5° hourly
   (b) maintain the room temperature at 37 °C
   (c) correct any dehydration urgently
   (d) administer thyroxine to correct levels

8 Which one of the following is the initial method of assessing a patient's level of consciousness? By:
   (a) monitoring their reaction to painful stimuli
   (b) testing limbs for movement or paralysis
   (c) checking their response to verbal stimuli
   (d) examining the pupillary reaction to light

9 Which of the following describes the function of the prostate gland:
   (a) production of spermatozoa
   (b) secretion of fluid to aid sperm mobility
   (c) prevention of bacteria entering the bladder
   (d) alteration of acidity in the urethra

10 Which one of the following is the effect of sudden cessation of corticosteroid therapy:
   (a) excessive glycosuria
   (b) severe hypertension
   (c) Cushing's syndrome symptoms
   (d) Addisonian type crisis

11 Which of the following is the best way to care for a patient suffering chronic pain:
   (a) administer prescribed analgesia at regular intervals
   (b) give analgesia whenever requested
   (c) offer to discuss their fears and worries with a minister
   (d) encourage activities and diversions

12 Which of the following is the reason tablets are enteric coated? In order that their contents do not:
   (a) cause an allergic reaction
   (b) irritate the gastric mucosa
   (c) dissolve until they reach the stomach
   (d) make the teeth become discoloured

13 Which one of the following is a common problem affecting patients receiving enteral nutrition:
   (a) diarrhoea
   (b) indigestion
   (c) overhydration
   (d) gastric distension

14 Which of the following is the reason why patients with liver disease suffer abdominal distension? Because:
   (a) nutrients are not fully metabolized
   (b) digestive juices build up in the intestines
   (c) capillary fluid passes into the abdominal cavity
   (d) peristalsis in the ileum is abnormal

15 Which of the following events occurs when blood clots:
   (a) lymphocytes increase in viscosity
   (b) thrombin is absorbed by erythrocytes
   (c) fibrinogen breaks down to release fibrin
   (d) corpuscles become trapped in the fibrous mesh

16 Which of the following observations would indicate that a patient was in a state of shock, pulse rate:
   (a) weak and slow, blood pressure rising
   (b) rapid and weak, skin colour pale
   (c) strong and slow, blood pressure falling
   (d) rapid and strong, skin colour flushed

17 Which one of the following actions should the nurse take if a patient receiving an intravenous infusion complains of breathlessness, palpitations and headache:
   (a) observe the respiratory rate half hourly
   (b) check the blood pressure
   (c) stop the infusion running
   (d) weigh the patient

18 Which of the following terms describes the process by which water molecules move from an area of low to high concentration through a semi-permeable membrane:
   (a) active transport
   (b) diffusion
   (c) cell respiration
   (d) osmosis

19 Which of the following is the correct method of catheter hygiene:
   (a) swab up and down with Savlon twice daily
   (b) use one cotton wool ball for around the urethra
   (c) swab away from the urethra with soap and water four hourly
   (d) use alcohol impregnated wipes and gloves around the urethra

20 Which one of the following actions should the nurse take if during a medicine round a patient prescribed a tablet complains of nausea:
   (a) administer the preparation intramuscularly

(b) ask the doctor to prescribe an anti-emetic
(c) miss out the tablet and dispense it later
(d) omit the drug, record and report the omission

21 Which of the following should the nurse advise a patient after a mastectomy before discharge home:
(a) to offer the affected arm for injections
(b) not to use the affected arm for heavy household duties
(c) to exercise the arm to its full range daily
(d) not to wear any tight fitting clothes

22 Which of the following is the secretory phase of the menstrual cycle? The period:
(a) prior to menstruation
(b) during follicle development
(c) prior to ovulation
(d) during progesterone secretion

23 Which of the following is the primary lesion of syphilis? A:
(a) chancre
(b) condylomata
(c) gumma
(d) gyrus

24 Which of the following amounts in millilitres of a solution containing 250 milligrams per millilitre should be drawn into the syringe to administer a dose of 62.5 milligrams:
(a) 0.025
(b) 0.25
(c) 2.5
(d) 12.5

25 Which one of the following is the correct procedure when wearing a gown for source isolation nursing:
(a) it should be hung with the clean side folded out
(b) should be laundered after single use
(c) only the clean side touches the uniform
(d) requires no special laundry identification

26 Which of the following substances initiates phagocytosis when it is released from injured cells:
(a) leukoplakia
(b) antibody
(c) fibrin
(d) histamine

27 Which of the following are patients suffering rheumatoid arthritis likely to demonstrate:
(a) no improvement after steroid therapy
(b) general malaise and swollen joints
(c) pain in the lumbar region
(d) increased joint mobility and flexibility

28 Which of the following is the problem most likely to affect patients suffering myasthenia gravis:
(a) difficulty with balance and positioning limbs
(b) loss of neuronal control of lower limbs
(c) muscle spasms and tenesmus at rest
(d) inability to sustain muscular effort

29 Which of the following numbers of 600 milligram tablets should be dispensed for a prescription of 1.8 grams:
(a) 3   (b) 4   (c) 5   (d) 6

Mrs Julie Smith is 45 years old, obese, mother of three children, who is to be admitted for a cholecystectomy and choledochotomy.

30 Which of the following explains why Mrs Smith complained of nausea, indigestion and pain after fatty foods? Because:
(a) saturated fats are difficult to digest
(b) bile was not entering the duodenum
(c) the liver was not producing bile
(d) she should not have eaten fatty foods

31 Which of the following symptoms would Mrs Smith also be likely to complain about:
  (a) dark urine, clay coloured stools, itchy skin
  (b) light urine, dark brown stools, yellow skin
  (c) straw coloured urine, putty coloured stools, yellow sclera
  (d) normal urine, brown stools, dry flaky skin

32 Which of the following explains why Mrs Smith may suffer respiratory problems after her operation, because:
  (a) she was overweight and did not exercise
  (b) she is anxious and may overbreathe
  (c) the incision is near the diaphragm
  (d) there was bile in the blood stream

33 Which one of the following is the reason the T-tube is clamped off for short periods after exploration of the common bile duct:
  (a) to prevent blockage and pain
  (b) to assess whether bile is entering the duodenum
  (c) to determine the amount of bile the liver is making
  (d) as an overflow valve

34 Which of the following actions should the nurse make if Mrs Smith's abdominal wound ruptured after removal of sutures:
  (a) apply steristrips and pad well
  (b) quickly cover with a sterile gauze swab
  (c) call the surgeon to resuture the wound
  (d) put a pressure bandage around her waist

Mr Peter East is a 55-year-old managing director, he is married with two children, aged 21 and 24 who are away at university. He is busy socially, playing squash and golf and he and his wife dine out frequently. He has been admitted with a diagnosis of myocardial infarction:

35 Which of the following describes myocardial infarction:
  (a) intense pain in the chest on inspiration relieved by rest
  (b) interruption of blood supply to cardiac muscle
  (c) irregular heart rhythm due to low blood pressure
  (d) due to massive vasodilatation of the coronary artery

36 Which one of the following is the reason Mr East would be prescribed diamorphine:
  (a) to avoid the problem of addiction
  (b) the problem of intolerance is unlikely
  (c) it depresses the vagus nerve
  (d) it blocks pain sensation

37 Which one of the following is the **most** important observation the nurse should make on Mr East:
  (a) pulse and blood pressure
  (b) temperature and respiratory rate
  (c) urinalysis and blood pressure
  (d) respiratory rate and skin colour

38 Mr East's condition deteriorates rapidly and he becomes cold and clammy. Which of the following is correct, blood pressure falls if:
  (a) control by the vasometer centre is lost
  (b) blood becomes more viscous
  (c) peripheral resistance is high
  (d) cardiac output is increased

His condition deteriorates further and a cardiac arrest is diagnosed.

39 Which of the following describes the priorities of resuscitation of a collapsed patient:
  (a) circulation, breathing, airway   (b) airway, circulation, breathing
  (c) breathing, airway, circulation   (d) airway, breathing, circulation

Mr Albert Long is a 55-year-old bricklayer, he is a bachelor and lives in digs. He smokes 20 cigarettes a day and drinks 3 pints of beer most nights. He has never been in hospital before. He was admitted as an emergency with a diagnosis of strangulated inguinal hernia, and had been vomiting faecal fluid for 6 hours. He is to go for surgery in 2 hours.

40 Which of the following observations would lead the nurse to suspect Mr Long is dehydrated:
  (a) wrinkled skin, bradycardia, hypertension, oliguria

(b) thirst, weight loss, hypertension, tachycardia
(c) dry mucous membranes, wrinkled skin, hypotension, bradycardia
(d) hypotension, weight loss, oliguria, tachycardia
41 Which of the following actions should the nurse take after passing a nasogastric tube:
  (a) aspirate and check the fluid with litmus paper
  (b) introduce a small amount of air into the tube before aspiration
  (c) aspirate the tube after introducing 30 ml of sterile water
  (d) lubricate the tube with olive oil before passing it
42 Which of the following describes the main principle of Mr Long's care:
  (a) ensure the right patient goes to theatre for the correct operation
  (b) check the surgeon's orders for preparation are completed correctly
  (c) instruct the patient how to breathe deeply and move limbs postoperatively
  (d) prepare the patient psychologically and physically for the operative period
43 Which of the following problems is **most** likely to affect Mr Long after he regains consciousness following anaesthesia:
  (a) haemorrhage
  (b) lung congestion
  (c) pain and discomfort   **(d)** paralytic ileus or flatus

Mr John Smith is a 24-year-old university student who was admitted after collapsing on the football field. On admission he looks flushed and his breath smells of acetone.
44 Which one of the following is the reason a ketoacidotic coma occurs? Because of:
  (a) increased blood glucose level
  (b) decreased blood glucose level
  (c) increased protein digestion and ketone formation.
  (d) incomplete fat breakdown with excess acid formation
45 Which of the following describes the principles of John's treatment:
  (a) insulin therapy, urinalysis and specific gravity measurement, reducing diet
  (b) fluid restriction, insulin therapy, protein restriction, specific gravity measurement
  (c) urinalysis, carbohydrate control, insulin therapy, blood glucose analysis
  (d) blood glucose analysis, urinalysis, fluid restriction, carbohydrate control
46 Which of the following would be the **most** suitable plan for John's future:
  (a) teach him to administer his insulin and balance carbohydrates and exercise
  (b) show him a special diet sheet and get him to stick to it
  (c) inform John's general practitioner and ask him to go for check-ups
  (d) request the district nursing service to supervise John at home
47 After visiting time one evening, John complains of feeling weak and 'strange'. Which of the following actions should the nurse take:
  (a) ask John to rest on his bed
  (b) give John a glass of milk to drink
  (c) ask for a sample of urine to test
  (d) give the next dose of insulin immediately
48 Which of the following should the nurse stress when teaching John about his condition:
  (a) that he should not play football without extra insulin
  (b) that he should not try to lose weight
  (c) extra fluid may be needed if his urinalysis is positive
  (d) to alternate the site of his injection

Mrs Elsie Jones, 65 years old, an ex-headmistress now retired and divorced, suffered a cerebral thrombosis at home 2 days ago. On admission she was suffering right hemiplegia, aphasia and absent gag reflex.
49 Which of the following features would you expect Mrs Jones to develop? A paralysis which is:
  (a) spastic on the same side as the intracerebral lesion
  (b) flaccid on the opposite side to the intracerebral lesion
  (c) spastic on the opposite side to the intracerebral lesion
  (d) flaccid on the same side as the intracerebral lesion

50 Which of the following positions should Mrs Jones be nursed in:
   (a) semiprone
   (b) lateral
   (c) semi-recumbent
   (d) prone

51 Which of the following is the **most** important in preventing pressure sore development:
   (a) regular washing and careful drying
   (b) use of ripple mattress or air rings
   (c) regular change of position
   (d) use of sheepskins and bedcradles

52 Which one of the following actions should the nurse take if Mrs Jones' catheter becomes blocked and overflows:
   (a) perform catheter hygiene four hourly
   (b) check her bowel function each day
   (c) irrigate the catheter with water
   (d) change the catheter for a smaller one

Mandy Potter aged 8 years suffers from asthma. She has been admitted this time with an acute attack, her mother and father are with her.

53 Which of the following describes the problem Mandy is suffering:
   (a) muscular spasm in the bronchioles
   (b) increased carbon dioxide levels
   (c) hyperventilation associated with anxiety
   (d) inability to cough up tenacious sputum

54 Which of the following describes the aim of treatment for Mandy:
   (a) postural drainage and humidified oxygen
   (b) expanding the lumen of the bronchioles
   (c) controlling her anxiety state
   (d) reducing the pulmonary secretions

55 Which of the following actions should the nurse take when Mandy becomes upset and breathless when her parents are about to go home:
   (a) play hide and seek with her and let them slip away
   (b) explain that they will be back soon
   (c) ask them to ignore her behaviour as she is ill
   (d) request that one of them might stay overnight

56 Which of the following plans would be best for Mandy on her first morning in the ward:
   (a) rest on her bed playing with a jigsaw and books
   (b) to join the other children after a shower and hairwash
   (c) sit quietly by her bed until the physiotherapist calls
   (d) begin to walk about and meet the other children

Answers to practice test 1

1	(d)	29	(a)
2	(c)	30	(b)
3	(b)	31	(a)
4	(b)	32	(c)
5	(a)	33	(b)
6	(d)	34	(d)
7	(a)	35	(b)
8	(c)	36	(d)
9	(b)	37	(a)
10	(d)	38	(a)
11	(a)	39	(d)
12	(b)	40	(d)
13	(a)	41	(a)
14	(c)	42	(d)
15	(d)	43	(c)
16	(b)	44	(d)
17	(c)	45	(c)
18	(d)	46	(a)
19	(c)	47	(b)
20	(d)	48	(d)
21	(b)	49	(c)
22	(a)	50	(a)
23	(a)	51	(c)
24	(b)	52	(d)
25	(c)	53	(a)
26	(d)	54	(b)
27	(b)	55	(d)
28	(d)	56	(a)

Practice test 2

1 Which one of the following skills is most useful to the nurse when admitting a patient:
(a) clinical expertise
(b) teaching ability
(c) interpersonal communication
(d) problem identification

2 Which of the following is the correct position for the nurse to adopt when lifting a patient:
(a) feet close together and legs straight
(b) back straight and feet together
(c) feet wide apart and back straight
(d) back curved and feet wide apart

3 Which of the following are the cardinal signs of inflammation:
(a) pain, pus, redness, papilloedema, increased nerve supply
(b) heat, redness, pain, swelling, loss of function
(c) oedema, pus, pain, pallor, decreased white cell count
(d) redness, pain, swelling, heat, loss of sensation

4 Which of the following describes epilepsy:
(a) due to head injury or brain cell death
(b) an involuntary loss of consciousness
(c) due to occasional irregular brain waves
(d) an emotionally based nervous instability

5 On which of the following days of the menstrual cycle does ovulation normally occur:
(a) 10   (b) 14   (c) 24   (d) 28

6 Which of the following problems would cause most concern in a patient after a lumbar puncture:
(a) alteration in mental state
(b) dysuria and frequency
(c) tingling in the upper limbs
(d) headache and nausea

7 Which of the following parts of the heart does blood enter when returning from the lungs:
(a) left ventricle
(b) right ventricle
(c) left atrium
(d) right atrium

8 Which one of the following would occur in the male if no gonadotrophin was produced? Absence of:
(a) spermatozoa
(b) androgen
(c) testosterone
(d) libido

9 Which of the following is the reason a person attending casualty with a wound obtained while gardening would be prescribed anti-tetanus immunoglobulin:
(a) to stimulate antigen production
(b) for immediate protection by antibodies
(c) to provide a target for lymphocytes
(d) for increased active immunity

10 Which of the following is the reason patients are placed prone for half an hour four times daily after undergoing mid-thigh amputation? To:
(a) ensure optimum stump shape
(b) improve circulation in remaining tissue

(c) reduce stump oedema

(d) prevent flexion contractures

11 Which of the following plans would be **most** useful to a patient with a right side hemiparesis:

(a) active movement of limbs twice daily

(b) bilateral straight leg raising exercises

(c) full passive range of movements three times daily

(d) muscle strengthening exercises to right limbs

12 Which one of the following actions should the nurse take if she suspects a patient's wound has become infected:

(a) clean the wound with a bacteriocidal solution twice daily

(b) send a swab for bacteriological examination

(c) change the dressing aseptically

(d) observe the wound site daily

13 Into which of the following areas is the needle placed during a lumbar puncture:

(a) pia mater   **(b)** pyramidal tract   **(c)** solar plexus   **(d)** subarachnoid space

14 Which of the following is a carrier of a communicable disease? A person who:

(a) is asymptomatic but is incubating the disease

(b) has been in close proximity to an infected person

(c) is asymptomatic and transmits the disease

(d) has had the disease and is non-infectious

15 Which of the following observations would indicate rising intracranial pressure:

(a) increasing respiratory rate, decreasing pulse rate, rigors

(b) decreasing pulse rate, rising blood pressure, unequal pupils

(c) increasing blood pressure, decreasing respiratory rate, rigors

(d) decreasing pulse rate, rising respiratory rate, unequal pupils

16 For which of the following reasons is traction applied to a fractured lower limb? In order to:

(a) prevent over extension of the muscles

(b) avoid weightbearing and muscle strain

(c) elevate the limb in a neutral position

(d) pull the bone ends to maintain a position

17 Which one of the following problems would affect a patient with a prolapsed uterus:

(a) stress incontinence

(b) fundal pain

(c) vaginal cramp

(d) faecal impaction

18 Which of the following plans of care would most benefit a patient with dyspnoea due to congestive cardiac failure? Oxygen concentration:

(a) high and positioned with one pillow

(b) low and increase active movements

(c) high and improve blood volume

(d) low and positioned upright

19 Which one of the following is the maximum amount in millilitres that can be given by intramuscular injection:

(a) 1.5

(b) 2

(c) 5

(d) 7.5

20 Which of the following is the primary aim of nursing an unconscious patient:

(a) maintenance of an airway

(b) prevention of pressure sores

(c) monitoring of consciousness level

(d) provision of fluid and nutrients

21 Which of the following is the **most** important detail to check before administering a medicine? That the:

(a) patient's hospital number is written in ink

(b) prescribed medicine is available on the ward

(c) patient's hospital number complies with the identity band

(d) drug does not adversely affect the patient

22 Which of the following is the effect of an increase in circulating red blood cells:
   (a) reduced carbon dioxide content
   (b) greater blood viscosity
   (c) increased alkalinity
   (d) improved oxygen pressures

23 Which of the following actions should the nurse take if a diabetic patient complains of feeling faint and dizzy:
   (a) administer insulin on a sliding scale
   (b) obtain a specimen of urine for testing
   (c) give a glucose drink promptly
   (d) enquire about his activity level

24 Which of the following should the nurse advise a patient who developed signs of masculinity while on medication for Addison's disease:
   (a) explain how best to disguise the signs
   (b) explain it is a symptom of the disease
   (c) reassure her that the signs will disappear after the therapy
   (d) inform her that this is due to the therapy

25 Which one of the following statements is correct:
   (a) diarrhoea occurs due to loss of control of the coeliac muscles
   (b) decreased metabolism is associated with malabsorption syndrome
   (c) straining at stool is due to increased peristalsis
   (d) repeated failure to relax the external sphincter leads to constipation

26 Which of the following is the effect of high levels of circulating oestrogen:
   (a) ovulation occurs
   (b) reduction of follicle stimulating hormone
   (c) increase in ova production
   (d) lactation is stimulated

27 Which of the following observations would lead a nurse to think a patient is dehydrated:
   (a) absence of tears, weight loss, hypertension, oliguria
   (b) dysuria, hypotension, weight loss, thirst
   (c) hypertension, dry tongue, bradycardia, polyuria
   (d) tachycardia, weight loss, dry tongue, hypotension

28 Which of the following blood groups is the universal recipient:
   (a) AB
   (b) A
   (c) B
   (d) O

29 Which of the following describes the action of Glycerine suppositories? A(n):
   (a) faecal softener and lubricant
   (b) colonic irritant
   (c) bulk additive and stimulant
   (d) peristaltic regulator

Mr Derek Mann, aged 58, is a retired postman. He lives on a council estate with his wife and two teenage sons. Each year he suffers from acute attacks of breathlessness and wheezing, often followed by bouts of coughing producing copious sputum.

30 Mr Mann's dyspnoea is due to:
   (a) excess fibrous tissue
   (b) spasm of the smooth muscle
   (c) dilatation of the bronchi
   (d) inflammation of the bronchi

31 Which of the following describes the priority of Mr Mann's nursing care:
   (a) observe fluid balance accurately
   (b) assist to a position for easy breathing
   (c) promote hygiene and comfort
   (d) maintain observations of vital signs

32 Which of the following is the reason Mr Mann will be prescribed low oxygen percentages? Because he/his:
   (a) lung capacity is severely reduced
   (b) may overbreathe and exhale less carbon dioxide

    (c) breathing stimulus is low oxygen levels

    (d) may become used to the enriched air

33 Which of the following is most likely to help Mr Mann to expectorate:

    (a) postural drainage and suction four hourly

    (b) leaning forward on to padded bedtable

    (c) administration of codeine linctus

    (d) a fluid intake of 3 litres daily

34 Which of the following should the nurse advise Mr Mann before his discharge:

    (a) avoid crowds and outings in damp weather

    (b) take antibiotics over the winter period

    (c) keep the house temperature at 70°F (21°C) and wear woollen vests

    (d) ensure he is immunized against influenza each year

Mr Stewart is 59 and suffers congestive cardiac failure due to rheumatic heart disease. He is married with two children of 24 and 29 both of whom are married and live away from home.

35 Which of the following problems is **most** likely to be affecting Mr Stewart:

    (a) palpitations, dehydration and muscle weakness

    (b) dyspnoea, oedema and tiredness

    (c) oedema, dry mucous membranes and palpitations

    (d) nausea, loss of weight, oedema

36 Which of the following is the reason personal hygiene and pressure area care is a priority for Mr Stewart:

    (a) to remove bacteria from his skin

    (b) so that his limbs are repositioned regularly

    (c) promotes venous return and prevents stasis

    (d) to maintain the unbroken condition of his skin

37 Which of the following positions would Mr Stewart be nursed in whilst in bed:

    (a) dorsal recumbent to assist venous return

    (b) semi-recumbent for easy ventilation

    (c) semi-prone to preserve an airway

    (d) upright for reduction of pulmonary oedema

38 Which of the following is the principle of caring for a patient receiving diuretic drugs:

    (a) ensure diuretics are only administered in the morning

    (b) reduce the amount of salt and fluid intake

    (c) record the patient's weight daily

    (d) monitor the output accurately

39 Which of the following is the nurse's **main** responsibility when administering digoxin to a patient:

    (a) checking that the timing and quantity is correctly prescribed

    (b) observing the effect on the patient's condition

    (c) stopping the drug if the pulse rate is under 60

    (d) measuring the input and output accurately

Miss Ellen West is a spinster, aged 62 years, who has been admitted for three days before permanent sigmoid colostomy due to carcinoma of the colon.

40 Which of the following is the main function of the colon:

    (a) secretion of vitamins B and K   **(b)** breakdown of amino acids

    (c) absorption of water   **(d)** formation of gases

41 Which of the following is true? A colostomy in the descending colon:

    (a) will function throughout the night and day

    (b) will inevitably produce odour from the bag

    (c) should have a 3 cm space around the stoma

    (d) should be cleaned with soap and water

42 Which of the following actions should the nurse take if while performing a colonic washout, the patient complains of cramp:

    (a) ask him or her to turn into a recumbent position

    (b) stop the irrigation until the feeling goes

    (c) request that he or she tries to hold the fluid longer

    (d) hold the funnel higher to speed up the procedure

The night before Miss West's operation, the nurse notices she is pale and is sitting very quietly beside her bed.

43 Which of the following actions should the nurse take:
   (a) leave her alone to get some rest
   (b) sit down beside her and take time for discussion
   (c) ask her if she wants to ask any questions
   (d) explain about her operation again

Miss West recovers well from her operation.

44 Which of the following pieces of advice should the nurse give her before discharge:
   (a) to avoid swimming and going out to dinner frequently
   (b) eat plenty of fruit and continue playing golf carefully
   (c) change to a sedentary job and eat a high residue diet
   (d) to identify her own food tolerance and take moderate exercise

Miss Rita Clarke is 32 years old and has been admitted for re-assessment of her multiple sclerosis. She is unable to move independently or control her elimination.

45 Which of the following describes the characteristics of multiple sclerosis:
   (a) loss of myelin in patches throughout the nervous system
   (b) excessive electrical discharges in motor neurones
   (c) reduced chemical transmission at the synapses
   (d) loss of sensory neurone function below the spinal tract

46 Which of the following is the prognosis of this disease:
   (a) poor with terminal stages in weeks
   (b) good with the correct treatment regime
   (c) chronic with exacerbations and remissions
   (d) slow deterioration without remission

47 Which of the following is likely to be Miss Clarke's main nursing problem:
   (a) danger of skin breakdown
   (b) inability to maintain her own personal hygiene
   (c) danger of venous stasis or thrombosis
   (d) difficulty in breathing in and out freely

48 Which of the following sites would be most suitable for a subcutaneous injection of cyanocobalamin:
   (a) upper outer quadrant of the buttock
   (b) exterior aspect of the forearm
   (c) outer aspect of the thigh
   (d) into the abdominal wall

49 Which of the following referrals would be of most use to Miss Clarke when she goes home? To the:
   (a) home help organizer   (b) meals on wheels
   (c) district nursing service   (d) health visiting service

Mrs Ann Brown, aged 34, is married with a 3-year-old son. She and her husband run a grocer's shop. She is to be admitted for thyroidectomy.

50 Which of the following problems is **most** likely to be affecting Mrs Brown:
   (a) intolerance of heat
   (b) slow and irregular heart beats
   (c) nausea and vomiting
   (d) mental and physical tiredness

51 Which one of the following is the reason Mrs Brown's pulse will be checked when she is asleep? In order to:
   (a) check against her postoperative observations
   (b) establish the true base line recording
   (c) determine what her metabolic rate is at night
   (d) compare with recordings in the day

You find Mrs Brown in the bathroom crying after visiting time on her preoperative evening.

52 Which of the following actions should the nurse take:
   (a) ask her what she is crying for

(b) reassure her that she is in experienced hands

(c) let her explain what the trouble is in her own time

(d) make her a milky drink and give her night sedation early

53 Which of the following actions should the nurse take **first** if Mrs Brown becomes cyanosed and dyspnoeic while recovering from her anaesthetic:

(a) sit her up and check the suture line

(b) give low percentage oxygen via a ventmask

(c) remove the clips from the wound immediately

(d) replace the artificial airway and apply suction

54 Which of the following is the reason why Mrs Brown's clips will be removed, after 48–72 hours? To:

(a) prevent pressure behind the suture line

(b) minimize the extent of the scar

(c) reduce the difficulty experienced while swallowing

(d) allow freer movement of the neck`

Peter James, aged 30, is a solicitor, married with no children. He enjoys playing squash and rugby. He was admitted to your ward from casualty with a diagnosis of renal calculi and ureteric colic.

55 Which of the following describes the main principle of Peter's immediate care:

(a) recording blood pressure and pulse to assess shock

(b) sieve all urine to detect stones if passed

(c) regular administration of analgesia to control pain

(d) measuring fluid balance to monitor renal function

56 Which of the following results would you expect from an analysis of Peter's urine:

(a) haematuria, proteinuria, specific gravity 1.025

(b) specific gravity 1.005, haematuria, ketonuria

(c) ketonuria, specific gravity 1.005, decreased viscosity

(d) proteinuria, increased viscosity, specific gravity 1.025

57 Which of the following analgesics would benefit Peter most:

(a) pethidine 75 mg

(b) diamorphine 10 mg

(c) acetylsalicylic acid 600 mg

(d) dihydrocodeine tartrate 30 mg

58 Peter undergoes pyelolithotomy. Which of the following problems is most likely to trouble him postoperatively:

(a) inability to pass urine

(b) enuresis and flank pain

(c) burning and frequency

(d) difficulty in controlling sphincters

Peter was found to have calcium oxalate stones and was advised to take a low calcium diet.

59 Which of the following would Peter be best advised to select from the menu:

(a) chocolate pudding and custard

(b) vanilla ice cream with chocolate syrup and nuts

(c) tuna fish pie and cheese sauce

(d) roast beef, baked potatoes and sprouts

Answers to practice test 2

1	(c)	31	(b)
2	(c)	32	(c)
3	(b)	33	(d)
4	(c)	34	(a)
5	(b)	35	(b)
6	(a)	36	(d)
7	(c)	37	(b)
8	(a)	38	(c)
9	(b)	39	(c)
10	(d)	40	(c)
11	(c)	41	(d)
12	(b)	42	(b)
13	(d)	43	(b)
14	(c)	44	(d)
15	(b)	45	(a)
16	(d)	46	(c)
17	(a)	47	(a)
18	(d)	48	(c)
19	(c)	49	(c)
20	(a)	50	(a)
21	(c)	51	(d)
22	(b)	52	(c)
23	(c)	53	(a)
24	(c)	54	(b)
25	(d)	55	(d)
26	(b)	56	(a)
27	(d)	57	(a)
28	(a)	58	(c)
29	(a)	59	(d)
30	(d)		

Section V
Appendix

Units of quantity

Pressure	
millimetres of mercury (mm Hg)	kilopascals (kPa)
1	0.13
10	1.33
20	2.67
30	4.00
40	5.33
50	6.67
60	8.00
70	9.33
80	10.67
90	12.00
100	13.33
110	14.67
120	16.00
130	17.33
140	18.67
150	20.00

Table V.1 Units of pressure

Energy	
Calories (Cal)	kilojoules (kJ)
10	42
100	420
200	840
300	1260
400	1670
500	2090
600	2510
700	2930
800	3350
900	3770
1000	4190
2000	8370
3000	12560

1 Calorie (kilocalorie) = 1000 calories
= 4.18 kilojoules
= 0.0042 megajoules

Table V.2 Units of energy

Normal haematological values for adults

	Red cells	Haemoglobin	Packed cell volume (PCV, haematocrit)
Males	$5.5 \pm 1.0 \times 10^{12}/l$	15.5 ± 2.5 g/dl	0.47 ± 0.07
Females	$4.8 \pm 1.0 \times 10^{12}/l$	14.0 ± 2.5 g/dl	0.42 ± 0.05

Mean corpuscular volume (MCV)	85 ± 8 fl
Mean corpuscular haemoglobin (MCH)	29.5 ± 2.5 pg
Mean corpuscular haemoglobin concentration (MCHC)	33 ± 2 g/dl
Reticulocytes	0.2 to 2.0%
Leucocytes	$7.5 \pm 3.55 \times 10^9/l$

Tables V.3 and **V.4** Haematological values

Differential leucocyte count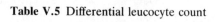

	%	× 10⁹/l	Miscellaneous units
Neutrophils	40 to 75	2.0 to 7.5	
Lymphocytes	20 to 45	1.5 to 4.0	
Monocytes	2 to 10	0.2 to 0.8	
Eosinophils	1 to 6	0.04 to 0.40	
Basophils	under 1	up to 0.1	
Platelets		150 to 400	
Prothrombin time, one stage			11 to 13 seconds
Prothrombin consumption index	up to 30		
Plasma fibrinogen			2.0 to 4.0 g/l
Cold agglutinin titre (4°C)			less than 64
Heterophile (anti-sheep red cell) agglutinin titre			less than 80
Heterophile (anti-sheep red cell) agglutinin titre (after absorption with guinea pig kidney)			less than 10
Plasma haemoglobin			10 to 40 mg/l
Red cell folate			160 to 640 µg/l
Serum vitamin B₁₂			160 to 925 µg/l
Sedimentation rate (westergreen 1h) at 30 ± 3°C			0 to 5 mm (males) 0 to 7 mm (females)

Table V.5 Differential leucocyte count

Normal biochemical values for adults

Serum or plasma

Cholesterol	3.6 to 7.2 mmol/l
Cortisol	170 to 720 nmol/l
Glucose (blood) fasting	3.3 to 5.6 mmol/l
random	3.3 to 8.4 mmol/l
Haptoglobin	0.3 to 2.0 g/l
Immunoglobins IgG	6.0 to 15.0 g/l
IgA	1.0 to 4.25 g/l
IgM	0.45 to 1.5 g/l
Iron	12 to 26 µmol/l
Total iron binding capacity	45 to 70 µmol/l
Lactate	550 to 1650 µmol/l
Lipoproteins (fasting)	
chylomicrons (L)	up to 0.28 g/l
pre-beta (M)	up to 2.4 g/l
beta (S)	up to 5.5 g/l
Magnesium	0.6 to 1.0 mmol/l
Osmolality	275 to 295 mmol/kg
Pyruvate	35 to 80 µmol/l
Thyroxine (T₄)	55 to 130 nmol/l
Urate	0.17 to 0.48 mmol/l (males) 0.14 to 0.39 mmol/l (females)

Table V.6 Normal serum or plasma values

Serum enzymes

Acid phosphatase	0.13 to 0.56 IU/l
Alkaline phosphatase	25 to 100 IU/l
Amylase	70 to 300 IU/l
ALT (GPT)	5 to 40 IU/l
AST (GOT)	5 to 45 IU/l
Creatine kinase (CK)	up to 80 IU/l
γ-Glutamyl transpeptidase (γ-GT)	up to 65 IU/l
Hydroxybutyrate dehydrogenase	up to 200 IU/l
Lactate dehydrogenase (LDH)	200 to 500 IU/l
Lipase	up to 1.5 units

Table V.7 Serum enzymes

Acidity/basicity

Plasma pH	7.36 to 7.44
P_{CO_2}	34 to 45 mm Hg
Standard bicarbonate (plasma)	2.15 to 25.0 mmol/l
Base excess	-2.3 to $+2.3$ mmol/l (males)
	-3.0 to $+1.6$ mmol/l (females)

Table V.8 Acidity/basicity

Cerebrospinal fluid

Glucose	2.0 to 4.5 mmol/l
Total protein	0.15 to 0.45 g/l
Globulin (qualitative)	no increase
IgG percentage of total protein	up to 13%
Lange curve	change up to 1

Table V.9 Cerebrospinal fluid values

Basic carbohydrate and calorie table

Food	Approximate weight or volume	Calories	Grams of carbohydrate
Beverages			
Coffee (white without sugar)	1 cup	15	–
Tea (white without sugar)	1 cup	15	–
Bread			
White	25 g (1 slice)	65	15
Wholemeal	25 g (1 slice)	50	10
Dairy products			
Butter	25 g	210	–
Cheese, Cheddar	25 g	120	–
Cream, single	2 tbs	45	1
Egg	one	80	
Milk, whole	1 cup	130	10
Drinks (alcoholic)			
Beer, draught	½ pint	100	10
Brandy	24 ml (measure)	55	–
Lager, draught	½ pint	135	10
Wine, dry	113 ml (glass)	75 – 100	–
Whisky, Scotch	24 ml (measure)	55	–
Fruit			
Apple	one, large	80	20
Banana	one, medium	80	20
Grapefruit	one, large	45	10
Orange	one, large	40	10
Pear	one, large	40	10
Meat, fish and poultry			
Bacon, lean, grilled	one rasher	75	–
Fish, white, raw	100 g	80	–
Meat, lean, cooked	100 g	160	–
Poultry, lean, white meat	100 g	140	–
Salmon, canned	100 g	155	–
Sausages, thick	two	400	10
Vegetables			
Carrots	½ cup	25	5
Peas, fresh	½ cup	55	10
Potatoes, boiled	50 g	40	10
Sweetcorn	5 tbs	45	10

Table V.10 Basic carbohydrate and calorie chart

Recommended energy intakes for average heights and weights

Category	Age (years)	Weight (kg)	Height (m)	Energy needs (Cal)	(MJ)
Male	11 – 14	45	157	2700	11.3
	15 – 18	66	176	2800	11.8
	19 – 22	70	177	2900	12.2
	23 – 50	70	178	2700	11.3
	51 – 75	70	178	2400	10.1
	76 +	70	178	2050	8.6
Female	11 – 14	46	157	2200	9.2
	15 – 18	55	163	2100	8.8
	19 – 22	55	163	2100	8.8
	23 – 50	55	163	2000	8.4
	51 – 75	55	163	1800	7.6
	76 +	55	163	1600	6.7

Table V.11 Recommended energy intakes for average heights and weights

Energy expenditure for various activities

Activity	Calories per hour
Sedentary reading, writing, eating, watching television, sewing, typing; activities done sitting down with little or no arm movement.	80 to 100
Light cooking, washing up, dusting, ironing, walking slowly; activities done standing requiring some arm movement or sitting which are more strenuous.	110 to 160
Moderate making beds, mopping, scrubbing, sweeping, light polishing, light gardening, moderately fast walking; activities done standing requiring moderate arm movement or sitting requiring more vigorous arm movement.	170 to 240
Vigorous heavy scrubbing, washing by hand, making beds, walking fast, bowling, golfing, gardening, other heavy work.	250 to 350
Strenuous swimming, playing tennis, running, cycling, dancing, football.	350 and over

Table V.12 Energy expenditure for various activities

Priming the set

1 Insert the piercing needle into the fluid container in the normal manner and prime the set.
2 Tape the stopcock to the IV stand below the level of the patient's atrium. Tape the upper end of the manometer tube to the IV stand. The manometer tube should be taut.
3 Adjust the stopcock to position 3 and half fill the manometer tube. Close the roller clamp and return stopcock to position 2.
4 Remove the tip protector of distal end of the set and expel the air from the tubing by opening the roller clamp. Connect set to needle/catheter.
5 Stick the self adhesive scale to the IV stand so that the zero mark on the scale corresponds with the level of the right atrium.

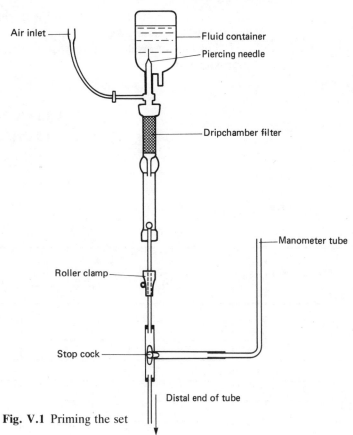

Fig. V.1 Priming the set

A TYPICAL INTRAVENOUS FLUID PRESCRIPTION CHART				Name Record No.					
Date	Intravenous Fluid and Additives to bag/bottle not bolus injections	Vol	Regime	Doctor's Signature	Time Started	Time Finished	Container Batch No	Nurse's Signature

Chart V.1 Intravenous fluid prescription chart

Care of the CVP line

1 Site of insertion inspected daily for signs of infection which should be reported.
2 Manometer line must always be well filled with fluid to avoid possibility of air embolism.
3 CVP set and fluid should be changed daily.

If infection is avoided CVP line may remain in situ for weeks.

Complications which may occur

1 Air embolism
2 Pneumothorax
   Hydrothorax – IV fluid in pleural cavity
   Haemothorax
   Infection

Removal of CVP line

This must be carried out slowly and with care. Any change occurring in patient's condition during removal should be noted and reported.

Following removal of the catheter, pressure should be applied to the site of entry for approximately 5 minutes

A TYPICAL
FLUID CHART

(For use of Nursing Staff)

Record No.

NAME .... WARD .... SHEET No. ....

1. A red line is drawn across the page at the end of each 24 hours.
2. All measurements in ml. (cc.).
3. English numerals only to be used.

Date	Time	Initials of Nurse	INTAKE					OUTPUT.					Time	Initials of Nurse
			Nature of Fluid	ROUTE		ml. left	Suc-tion	Diarr-hœa	Vomit	Drain-age	URINE		
				Mouth	I.V.									

Chart V.2 Fluid balance chart

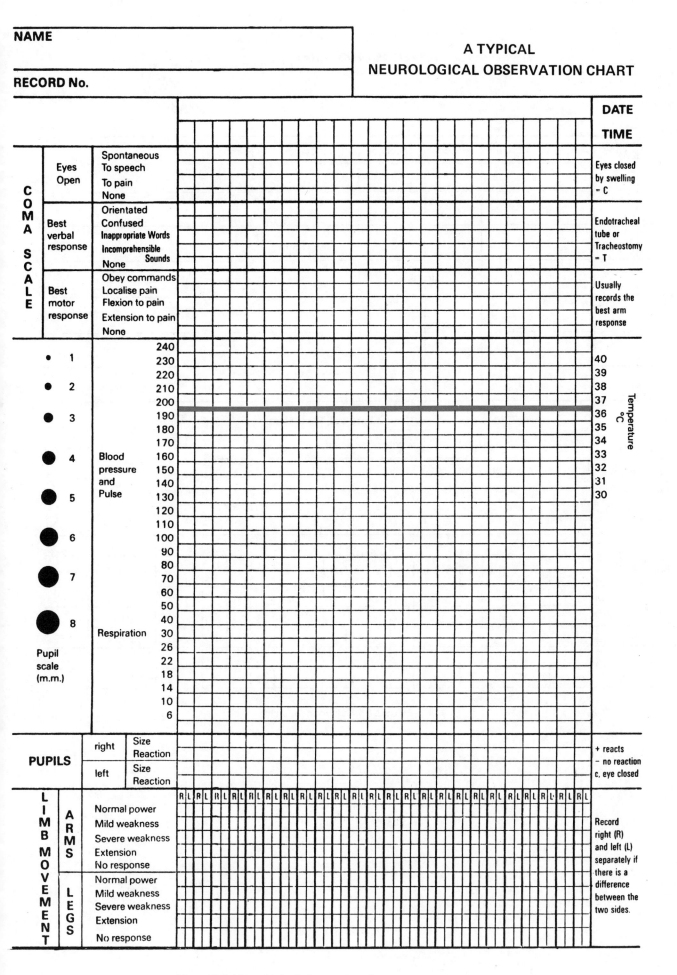

Chart V.3 Neurological observation chart

A TYPICAL STOOL CHART

NAME: **WARD:**

Date	Time	Amount	Colour	Blood	Mucous	Consistency	Remarks

Chart V.4 Stool chart

A CONTINENCE CHART

■ — Continent asked for aid (bedpan, urinal, commode toilet)
▲ — Continent only when offered aid (bedpan, urinal, commode toilet)
O — Aid given same not used
R — Aid offered but refused

U — Incontinent of urine
F — Incontinent of faeces
✓ — Dry
X — Damp/Dribble

	Morning				Afternoon				Evening				Night											
Date	9	10	11	12	1	2	3	4	5	6	7	8	9	10	11	12	1	2	3	4	5	6	7	8	Comments

Chart V.5 Continence chart

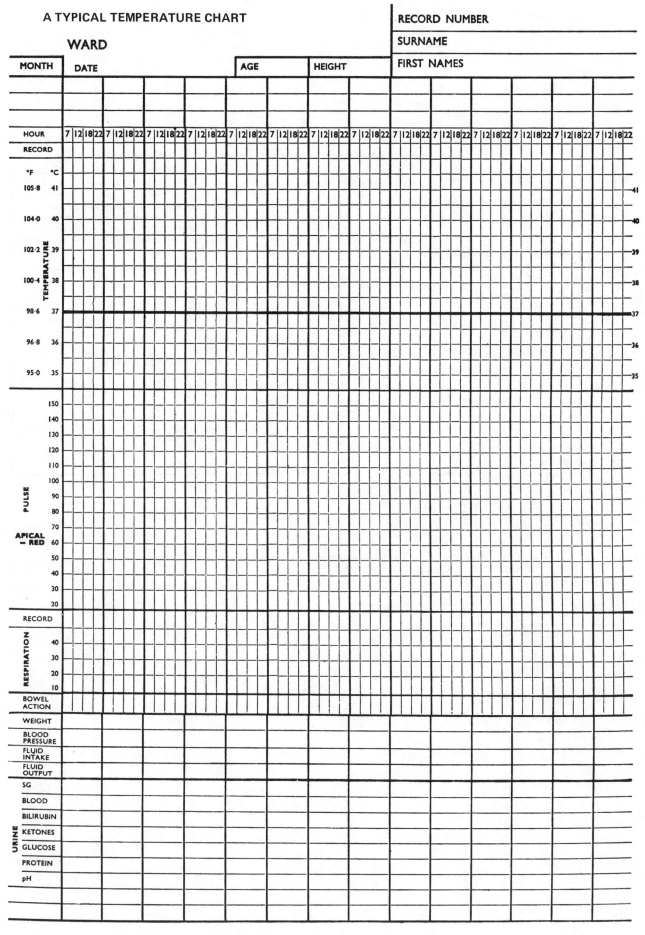

Chart V.6 Temperature chart

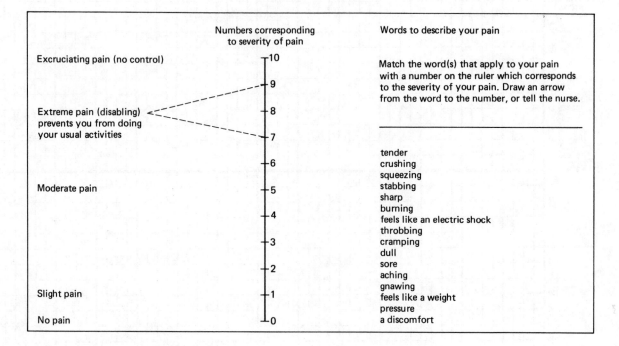

Fig. V.2 The pain ruler

Source: Bourbonnais, F., 'Pain assessment: development of a tool for the nurse and the patient' (*Journal of Advanced Nursing*, 6, 277–282, 1981).

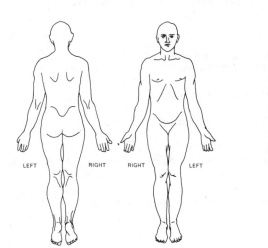

Excruciating	5
Very severe	4
Severe	3
Moderate	2
Just noticeable	1
No pain at all	0
Patient sleeping	S

PAIN OBSERVATION CHART

PATIENT
IDENTIFICATION
LABEL

DATE . . . .

SHEET NUMBER . . . .

TIME	PAIN RATING										MEASURES TO RELIEVE PAIN Specify where starred									COMMENTS FROM PATIENTS AND/OR STAFF	Initials
	BY SITES								OVER- ALL	ANALGESIC GIVEN (Name, dose, route, time)	Lifting	Turning	Massage	Distracting activities*	Position change*	Additional aids*	Other*			
	A	B	C	D	E	F	G	H												

THIS CHART records where a patient's pain is and how bad it is, by the nurse asking the patient at regular intervals. If analgesics are being given regularly, make an observation *with* each dose and another *half-way between* each dose. If analgesics are given only 'as required', observe two-hourly. When the observations are stable and the patient is comfortable, any regular time interval between observations may be chosen.

TO USE THIS CHART ask the patient to mark all his or her pains on the body diagram above. Label each site of pain with a letter (ie. A, B, C etc.)

Then at each observation time ask the patient to assess:
1   the pain in each separate site since the last observation. Use the scale above the body diagram, and enter the number or letter in the appropriate column.
2   the pain overall since the last observation. Use the same scale and enter in column marked OVERALL.

Next, record what has been done to relieve pain:
3   note any analgesic given since the last observation — stating name, dose, route, and time given.
4   tick any other nursing care or action taken to ease pain.

Finally, note any comment on pain from patient or nurse (use the back of the chart as well, if necessary) and initial the record.

Chart V.7 The pain chart

Reproduced by permission of Jennifer Raiman, The London Hospital Medical College.

THE NORTON SCORING SCALE FOR PRESSURE SORE RISK CALCULATION

Instructions

1. Choose the most appropriate description of the patient (1, 2, 3 or 4)
   under each of the five headings (A to E) and total the result.

2. Record the score and date in the patient's notes or on the chart.

3. Assess weekly and whenever there is any change in the patient's condition
   and/or circumstances of care.

A score of 14 or below denotes a need for intensive care, i.e. 1-2 hourly changes of position and the use of pressure-relieving aids.

Note: When oedema of the sacral area has been present, a rise above 14
does not indicate less risk of a lesion.

SCORING SYSTEM: TOTAL SCORE OF 14 AND BELOW — 'AT RISK'

		A Physical condition	B Mental condition	C Activity	D Mobility	E Incontinent
		Good 4	Alert 4	Ambulant 4	Full 4	Not 4
		Fair 3	Apathetic 3	Walk/Help 3	Slightly limited 3	Occasionally 3
		Poor 2	Confused 2	Chairbound 2	Very limited 2	Usually/ Urine 2
Patient's name	Date	Very bad 1	Stuporous 1	Bedfast 1	Immobile 1	Doubly 1

Chart V.8 The Norton scoring scale for pressure sore risk calculation

Source: Norton, D., McLaren R. and Exon-Smith, A. N., *An investigation of geriatric nursing problems in hospital* (London, National Corporation for the Care of Old People, 1962, reprinted by Churchill Livingstone, Edinburgh, 1975). Reproduced by permission of NCCOP.

CODE OF PROFESSIONAL CONDUCT
FOR THE NURSE, MIDWIFE AND HEALTH VISITOR UKCC 1984

Each registered nurse, midwife and health visitor shall act, at all times, in such a manner as to justify public trust and confidence, to uphold and enhance the good standing and reputation of the profession, to serve the interests of society, and above all to safeguard the interests of individual patients and clients.

Each registered nurse, midwife and health visitor is accountable for his or her practice, and, in the exercise of professional accountability shall:

1 Act always in such a way as to promote and safeguard the well being and interests of patients/clients.

2 Ensure that no action or omission on his/her part or within his/her sphere of influence is detrimental to the condition or safety of patients/clients.

3 Take every reasonable opportunity to maintain and improve professional knowledge and competence.

4 Acknowledge any limitations of competence and refuse in such cases to accept delegated functions without first having received instruction in regard to those functions and having been assessed as competent.

5 Work in a collaborative and co-operative manner with other health care professionals and recognise and respect their particular contributions within the health care team.

6 Take account of the customs, values and spiritual beliefs of patients/clients.

7 Make known to an appropriate person or authority any conscientious objection which may be relative to professional practice.

8 Avoid any abuse of the privileged relationship which exists with patients/clients and of the privileged access allowed to their property, residence or workplace.

9 Respect confidential information obtained in the course of professional practice and refrain from disclosing such information without the consent of the patient/client, or a person entitled to act on his/her behalf, except where disclosure is required by law or by the order of a court or is necessary in the public interest.

10 Have regard to the environment of care and its physical, psychological and social effects on patients/clients, and also to the adequacy of resources, and make known to appropriate persons or authorities any circumstances which could place patients/clients in jeopardy or which militate against safe standards of practice.

11 Have regard to the workload of and the pressures on professional colleagues and subordinates and take appropriate action if these are seen to be such as to constitute abuse of the individual practitioner and/or to jeopardise safe standards of practice.

12 In the context of the individual's own knowledge, experience, and sphere of authority, assist peers and subordinates to develop professional competence in accordance with their needs.

13 Refuse to accept any gift, favour or hospitality which might be interpreted as seeking to exert undue influence to obtain preferential consideration.

14 Avoid the use of professional qualifications in the promotion of commercial products in order not to compromise the independence of professional judgement on which patients/clients rely.

Reproduced by permission of the United Kingdom Central Council for Nursing, Midwifery and Health Visiting.

NOTES TO TUTORS AND TRAINERS

WHY DO WE ASK QUESTIONS?

1 Recall questions
  (a) To determine the extent of pre-knowledge.
  (b) To assess learning that has taken place and reinforce learner's sense of achievement.
  (c) As ice-breakers and openers, e.g. selection interviews.
  (d) To re-establish shared knowledge and experience.
  (e) To diagnose.

2 Process questions
  (a) To encourage the respondent to think more deeply.
  (b) To invite the giving of opinions, interpretation, analysis, etc.
    N.B. Frequently there is no one 'correct' answer. These questions can seldom be answered in one or two words.

3 Closed questions
  (a) To open a conversation.
  (b) To structure and control.
  (c) To gain factual information.
  (d) In assessment interviews.
  (e) To re-focus and clarify the issue.

4 Open questions
  (a) To give freedom and choice of response.
  (b) To explore a wide range of areas, e.g. counselling interviews.

5 Affective
  (a) To initiate recognition of feelings and attitudes.
  (b) To give freedom to discuss emotions.
  (c) To discuss reasons for these feelings and attitudes.

6 Leading
  (a) To stimulate the respondent towards a response expected by the initiator **and** the respondent.
  (b) To encourage the respondent to give an answer the questioner expects.
  (c) To emphasise the point of view of the questioner and elicit agreement from the respondent.

7 Rhetorical
  (a) To stimulate interest in the presentation.
  (b) To state or re-state a point.

8 Accusatory
  (a) To relieve the questioner's own feelings.
  (b) To require the respondent to justify himself.

9 Probing or follow-up
  (a) To elicit a clearer response.
  (b) To give the respondent an opportunity to re-assess and re-phrase.
  (c) To require respondents to make vague statements, specific.
  (d) To encourage the respondent to supply further information.
  (e) To give the respondent an opportunity to check back and reflect on the initial response.
  (f) To encourage the respondent to continue, and to maintain social inter-action.
      N.B. These echo probes are often non-verbal, e.g. para-language, eye contact, touch, pauses.
  (g) To give an opportunity for members of a group to express individual opinions. To evaluate the degree of consensus in a group.

10 Multiple
  (a) To attempt to get some form of answer where time is limited, e.g. radio and television interviews.
      N.B. These questions are often wasteful and confusing.

ASKING AND ANSWERING QUESTIONS

1 Why do we ask questions?
  (a) For information
  (b) For invitation
  (c) For requests
  (d) For encouragement
  (e) For persuasion
  (f) To initiate and maintain interaction

2 Form and function
  (a) Intonation is a question indicator.
  (b) The question form does not necessarily indicate a question.
  (c) We ask questions without using the question form.

Examples:

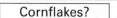
It's a lovely day today, isn't it?

Cornflakes?

How are you?

She did?

Yes?

Are all of these questions?
Which of them use the question form?
How is the fact that it is a question indicated?

3 Types of questions
  (a) *Closed questions*
  They are important for extracting facts and information quickly. They are only effective when the communicators have some shared knowledge and understanding of the purpose of the communication. They are worded to limit the range of answers. Closed questions can be irritating and confusing, especially when they are asked quickly and repetitively without reaction.

  Question: What is a suitable situation for the use of closed questions?
  (b) *Open questions*
      They are designed to encourage the respondent to answer as he wishes. However, to be

effective, they must be sincere, and time for a considered response must be given. They are too often asked as a ritual and answered by the questioner himself. "How are you? All right? That's good."

Question: What open questions do many nurses use as habit or ritual?

(c) *Choice questions*

Either/or. These can be used to force a respondent to choose one of two alternatives. It is, of course, quite possible that neither alternative would be the real choice of the respondent.

(d) *Negative questions* are 'loaded' to make negative responses less likely. They are useful in persuasion.

(e) *Leading questions* have the effect of blocking communication. They are phrased to get a response the questioner wants rather than a response the respondent might like to give.

(f) *Echoed questions/reflection*

Here are examples of different types of questions:

(1) Wouldn't you like to get into bed now?

(2) What would you like to do now?

(3) Are you cold?

(4) Which would you rather have, chocolate or Bovril?

(5) You don't want anything to eat, do you?

What kind of questions are they?

Why were they asked?

THE SKILL OF QUESTIONING
WORKSHEET 1

1 Statement: Questioning is involved in almost every form of social interaction because we use questions for such a variety of reasons.

2 Activity: Study this list of examples of reasons:

(1) to get factual information

(2) to find out how much other people know; to test

(3) to discover how people feel and what they think

(4) to stimulate interest

(5) to diagnose difficulties and problems

(6) to show interest in others

(7) to initiate an interaction

(8) encourage thought and revelation of ideas

(9) encourage self-determination and personal decision-making

(10) invite

(11) suggest a course of action

(12) disagree politely

(13) change the subject

(14) influence behaviour

(15) seek help

(16) motivate and maintain interest

(17) terminate interpersonal interaction

(18) deny responsibility

3 Task: Decide which of the examples should be tackled by individual members of your group. If there are problems, ask for help from a facilitator.

Practise working as an individual within a group. Only ask for help if other group members are free to answer.

Report your 'questions' to you group. Discuss whether or not they are accurate and appropriate.

Decide which examples you would like to present to the plenary group. If there are some you couldn't tackle, admit it and say why.

Discuss and decide the best method of presenting your task. You could:

begin with the examples you found impossible

give a visual example of question and answer

roll-play situations

ask members of other groups to participate

Decide **who** should be involved in the presentation.

4 Example: (1) To get factual information.
  Question: (1) What time does the train leave for Glasgow?
  Example: (7) To initiate an interaction.
  Question: (7) Haven't I met you before?

5 Activity: Present your conclusions to the plenary group.

WORKSHEET 2

Task: To examine the motives for questioning and the appropriacy of place, atmosphere, size of group and nature of question.

Statement: Some questions are self-interested; some are respondent-interested; others may have an element of both categories.

Examples: (1) 'Can you tell me which day is early closing?'
  (2) 'Shall I get you a hot water bottle?'
  (3) 'How would you like it if I made a pot of tea?'

Activity: Discuss:
  (1) which category these questions belong to
  (2) what the relationship of the questioner and respondent might be
  (3) the situation in which the questions could be asked

Statement: Some questions are more suitable in interpersonal communication; some are more appropriate in group interaction; some are acceptable and necessary in both situations. The place where questions are asked, the tone of voice in which they are asked, the number of people within earshot, the relative status of the questioner and respondent will all influence the attitude and the quality of the response.

Examples: (1) 'Can you tell me how you feel about the reduction of working hours?'
  (2) 'Would you take this bottle into the cubicle and give it to me when you've finished?'
  (3) 'You weren't born in this country, were you?'
  (4) 'Have you any idea why so many of our staff are often off sick?'
  (5) 'Why do you think we're having problems with the Nursing Process?'
  (6) 'Have you had your bowels open?'
  (7) 'How do you think we can cope with these cut-backs?'
  (8) 'Why were you late this morning?'
  (9) 'How do you feel about the prosthesis?'
  (10) 'Haven't you got any consideration for your colleagues?'

Activities: Study the questions

Discuss

(1) where and in what situations the questions are likely to be asked
(2) which of the 'interest' categories they belong to
(3) how many people are likely to be present
(4) how many people should be present
(5) whether the respondent can give an 'honest' answer in the situation

Decide

(1) what constraints would make it difficult to give an 'honest' answer.
(2) how the respondent might feel if forced to give an 'honest' answer.

Reproduced from *Communication for Care,* DHSS Project 1982, pp. 146–149.

Index

The main sections dealing with a subject are printed in bold.